Endoscopic Mitral Valve Surgery

Ralf Krakor

Endoscopic Mitral Valve Surgery

Handbook of Minimal-invasive Cardiac Surgery

Ralf Krakor

DE GRUYTER

Author
Ralf Krakor, MD
Klinikum Dortmund gGmbH
Klinik für Thorax-, Herz- und Gefäßchirurgie
Beurhausstr. 40
44137 Dortmund

ISBN 978-3-11-025422-8
e-ISBN 978-3-11-025445-7

Library of Congress Cataloging-in-Publication Data

Krakor, Ralf, 1963–
Endoscopic mitral valve surgery : handbook of minimal-invasive cardiac surgery / by Ralf Krakor.
p. ; cm.
ISBN 978-3-11-025422-8 (alk. paper)
1. Mitral valve—Surgery. 2. Heart—Surgery. 3. Endoscopic surgery. I. Title.
[DNLM: 1. Mitral Valve—surgery. 2. Cardiac Surgical Procedures—methods.
3. Endoscopy—methods. 4. Surgical Procedures, Minimally Invasive—methods.
WG 262]
RD598.K74 2011
617.4'120597–dc23 2011015403

Bibliographic information published by the Deutsche Nationalbibliothek
The Deutsche Nationalbibliothek lists this publication in the Deutsche Nationalbibliografie; detailed bibliographic data are available in the Internet at http://dnb.d-nb.de.

Typesetting: Apex CoVantage, LLC
Printing: Hubert & Co. GmbH & Co. KG, Göttingen
♾ Printed on acid-free paper
Printed in Germany
www.degruyter.com

Contents

Preface

The idea of writing this book came to me during a time of increasingly educational situations including discussions about endoscopic mitral valve surgery. In any event, it is the main result of an enjoyable evening of pleasant discussions in Prague during a two-day teaching session. At that time, I learned many things about myself and I was forced to reflect on my own reasons for the steps I took in endoscopic operations. In many situations it was basically clear to all of my colleagues how to carry out the main actions necessary for an endoscopic operation, and it seems to be very easy to repeat everything that they had seen at home. However, when it came to doing the same operation on their own, the limitations of just concentrating on the major things became often and very quickly apparent. As a result, many questions were repeated over several sessions. Another was observing the meaning of all those little things at the very beginning of endoscopic surgery.

With respect to all the colleagues who underwent the teaching and learning process for minimally invasive surgery, and as a support for everybody who would like to learn this wonderful kind of cardiac operation in the future, I have tried to arrange both the main things necessary for starting the operation and the little things that help achieve a positive result. I have tried to do this mostly without making general comments on the importance of mitral valve surgery or to the potential developments in general cardiac surgery. Beyond this, I believe it is very important to make some statements about the advantages of endoscopic mitral valve surgery and to make clear that this kind of operation is not just a passing fad. Instead, it has a permanent place among the various types of cardiac operations.

I would like to express my special thanks to Friedrich Mohr, who was my teacher for many years, to whom I owe the opportunity for unveiling the mysteries of endoscopic heart surgery.

It is also my sincere wish to thank all of my colleagues and coworkers for the support they have provided every day for performing genuinely satisfactory endoscopic procedures. It is a great pleasure for me to see how they are able to change an intricate procedure and specialized field into a routine and easygoing operation.

And, last but not least, I would like to thank all of my friends for their support and critical review of the text. A special thank counts to Romy, Hans, Fred, and Günter for a neverending readiness to help.

Dortmund, August 2011

Ralf Krakor

1 Introduction

1.1 General thoughts on endoscopic surgery

1.1.1 The philosophy

The ideas behind it

The goal of performing surgery on patients with structural defects of the mitral valve is reconstruction. Logically, this means preserving the native valve is an absolute priority, this being achieved via the access. Endoscopic access offers a number of benefits to the patient, although none of them are greater than the advantage of a reconstruction over valve replacement. If reconstruction seems to be too complex and the surgeon is (still) not sure that the reconstruction can be realized with the endoscopic access, the patient should be informed about the interrelation between the necessity of valve repair and the patient's prognosis before the operation starts. In that particular case, sternotomy should be the access of choice.

> The goal of the operation is reconstructing the valve. Access is only a means to an end.

It is expected that with growing experience these cases will become rare and it will be possible to reconstruct any defective valve using minimally invasive surgery. But at no point in time should the personal ambition of an individual take precedence over the safe reconstruction of heart valves.

Reconstruction of the mitral valve significantly increases the prognosis of the patients. This becomes especially clear when the operation is carried out before secondary damage is caused to the heart. At this early stage of the disease, patients are often asymptomatic, which is why they frequently disapprove of surgical intervention to a certain extent. A combination of endoscopic surgery and a full reconstruction of the valve can convince patients to be more likely to choose this procedure and therefore at least request an earlier date for the operation.

> A combination of valve reconstruction and endoscopic surgery makes an earlier operation possible, *which improves* patients' prognoses.

Here it seems necessary to give some background information about minimally invasive surgery. There is a wide range of terms in use for this field of surgery, most of which are synonymous: minimally invasive surgery, endoscopic mitral valve surgery, complete endoscopic surgery, minimally invasive heart surgery, and so on. It does not seem too important which term is used for this kind of operation. In the final analysis, it is the fundamental idea that represents a minimally invasive or at least a less traumatic operation. It should be obvious that the length of the incision is not the key criterion; it makes little difference to the patient whether a 15 or 20 cm long lateral thoracotomy or a sternotomy is performed. This is why we all should compromise on working atraumatically wherever feasible for a defined time period. This is the framework within which every surgeon will be able find the best way to apply his or her current skills and experience without increasing the risk for their patients. The idea of atraumatic access to the valve will spread with time and experience and people will focus on this agenda.

Complexity

The choice of endoscopic access will boost the complexity of the procedure many times over in comparison to conventionally performed operations.

In detail, endoscopic repair of the mitral valve consists of two complex procedures that have to mirror each other. Endoscopic access fundamentally differs from conventional surgery (such as being connected to the extracorporeal circulation, cardioplegia, and videoscopy) in that it requires precise work to just approach the valve, and is replete with multiple opportunities for making a mistake. These concerns do not inevitably endanger the patient or make the operation itself impracticable. However, in these situations the surgeon needs to focus more on managing complications than on the main goal of the operation. Therefore, one should get accustomed to a sequence of very purposeful routine processes that are relatively simple and can be applied to all patients.

The preparatory procedures should become routine, as simple as possible, and reproducible. The entire complexity of the procedure only requires a couple of easy steps.

The second part of repairing the valve itself might be relatively simple (e.g. quadrangular resection or implanting an artificial ring) or require greater experience and technical skills (e.g. implanting neochords or sliding plastic). This part of the operation may and will be more complicated because it is subordinate to the main goal, that is, reconstructing the valve (see Section 1.2.4 for further remarks on this issue).

These coherences make clear that the strategic orientation of endoscopic mitral valve reconstruction is to be understood and performed as a combination of a simple procedure for the access and a technically more demanding operation on the valve itself.

Experience

Nobody performs endoscopic surgery without having a feeling of entering new surgical territory, and this does not have anything to do with a person's surgical skills or experiences and is one reason why experienced surgeons have to show some staying power to acquire the experience needed.

Of course experience in the field of mitral valve repair is a prerequisite. The greater the experience the easier and faster a perfect combination of endoscopic approach and reconstruction of the valve can be achieved. However, more experience will only be acquired by using this procedure. The difference to the process of learning using a conventional access is only the access itself. If a surgeon has had his or her first experience with conventional mitral valve surgery and endoscopic access is his or her goal, then he or she should start to use the endoscopic technique soon. It seems to be easier to acquire knowledge in the field of endoscopic surgery parallel (the access and the repair technique) than to switch after a longer time from conventional surgery. Experience from conventional heart surgery shows that a transfer to endoscopic surgery is linked to certain limitations.

For team building and mutual support it is very useful to involve more than one surgeon into the process of learning this procedure. If there are two colleagues that develop a passion for minimally invasive mitral valve repair, the discussions about single steps, details, and mistakes can be very fruitful. And in case of complications it is always better to have two experienced surgeons than one.

> Experience from conventional heart surgery shows that a transfer to endoscopic surgery is linked to certain limitations. Existing extensive skills in the use of reconstructive techniques are advantageous, though.

Valve repair – frequency of valve replacements

A learning curve for every party involved is added to starting an endoscopic operation program with the goal to repair the mitral valve.

Certainly it is to be expected that, especially when the first patients are operated on successfully, a time with relative failures will follow and the rate of unsatisfactory results of valve repair will increase. This development often correlates with an expansion of indication and the acceptance of more complicated findings. At least the limitations of the existing skills will become apparent, but they will gradually subside with every new experience.

Therefore, this development is a necessary part of gaining experience in endoscopic surgery and must therefore absolutely be accepted. What is decisive is the critical reflection of unsatisfactory results and the absolute will to improve.

The consequence of valve insufficiency therapy is important for the acceptance of these interrelations also outside of the operation room. As a rule, valve replacement is always better than a bad reconstruction.

With a gain in training and experience the number of patients that get a valve replacement will decrease despite more complicated findings (▶Fig. 1.1).

> The primary goal is valve reconstruction. If this goal cannot be obtained the valve should be replaced with all consequences. Valve replacement is always better than a bad reconstruction.

1.1.2 The team

One of the most underestimated parts of endoscopic surgery is the quality of the teamwork among all staff members taking part in the operation. This means that all professional groups such as anesthesiologists, nurses, perfusionists, and, last but not least, surgical assistants know the goal of the operation and what it means for the patient.

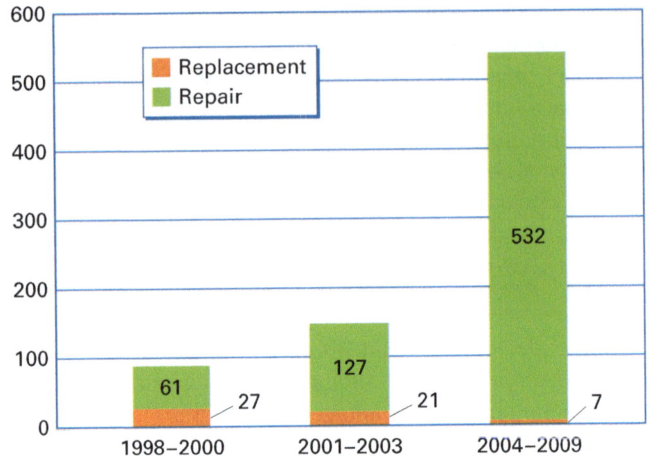

Fig. 1.1: Through a gain in experience and training and the consequent use of the method, a nearly complete rate of reconstruction can be achieved (author's own data, May 2009).

Whether the entire procedure turns out a success depends on the commitment to this idea of operation and the staff's capacity to work as a team.

At the beginning, a new operation is thrilling for everybody, leading to a readiness to accept more time-consuming operations and self-training. However, after several operations the appeal will wear off and sometimes an unsatisfactory result will call for an additional procedure, for example, a valve replacement might become due after a time-consuming repair (see also Section 1.1.1). At this point, it is absolutely necessary that the team around the surgeon supports the endoscopic procedure and knows that this is a normal development. It is very important that in such a situation the surgeon does not give up, and the staff members support a further operation.

The team is the key to success. Be sure that each staff member supports the main idea of the procedure – the endoscopic mitral valve repair.

Primarily at the first time, the high complexity of an endoscopic mitral valve repair leads to a situation where it is difficult for the surgeon to stay on top of things. It is very important that the surgeon trust all staff members to do their work. In other words – the best technical skills of a surgeon count for nothing if the basics of the procedure are unreliable, for example, the side-selected ventilation is not working, perfusion is too low, the nurse cannot handle the instruments, and so on. The development of an endoscopic program is up to every staff member and not to the surgeon alone.

1.1.3 Holding out

The reasons for performing endoscopic surgery are quite different: from the conviction that mitral valve repair is the best solution for the patient via the surgeon's personal ambition to the idea of an administration to get a more competitive heart surgical unit.

All of these interests focus on one thing: both the reliability and practicability of endoscopic mitral valve surgery have to be proven, not only once or twice but also in a serial and daily routine yielding satisfactory results.

The preparation of the staff takes time and a training program has to be completed. This includes not just a short medical round in a hospital with more experience in endoscopic mitral valve surgery. It means repeated training days at the hospital after more than one medical round, possibly for the whole staff, in experienced teams and implies certain efforts. Furthermore, investing in instruments and videoscopic equipment is expensive. These facts influence the situation of the surgeon who is responsible for the practical consequences of the endoscopic procedure (see also Section 1.2.1).

After the first successful procedures there will be a wide acceptance for introducing the new surgical method. But it will often be followed by one or two procedures with unsatisfactory results or a longer operation time (which may block the operation room for other procedures/other surgeons). When it becomes necessary to replace the valve after a long-lasting attempt to reconstruct it, enthusiasm may go down to zero. At this point the mental strength and the endurance of the surgeon are in demand. I would like to point out once more that it is easier to work together with a surgical colleague who has the same interest than alone.

Implementation and continuing endoscopic surgery needs endurance and mutual support even after complications have occurred.

The described situation is sometimes not easy to handle, but it is at least the only way for a successful implementation of an endoscopic surgical program.

1.2 How to start an endoscopic program

It is absolutely necessary that all partners involved in the introduction of this endoscopic procedure are aware of the cohesions described in the following chapters. Only when everybody from the management down to the nursing staff is convinced that it is right and necessary to introduce this procedure will the whole process be a success.

Today patients no longer accept that heart surgery should be connected to major stress events associated with the procedure. So we should no longer accept it either. Beside the (understandable) wish of the patients there is also a medical necessity to search for alternatives to classical heart surgery that is linked to median sternotomy, extracorporeal circulation, and major trauma. The patients we see today are often older and less healthy than they were 20 years ago (▶Fig. 1.2).

The result of this development is a significantly decreased tolerance of these patients against the trauma of open-heart surgery. After such a procedure, it often comes down to the physical reserves of the patient whether they recover quickly or rather slowly. Besides, the adaptation of the surgical intervention to the limited stress capacity of the older organism cannot be only a momentary solution; it describes the basic change of perspective. Even if the factor of limited stress capacity plays a rather subordinated role for younger patients, a similar necessity arises from the change of the social claim in this subgroup (see Section 1.2.2, Cosmetic reason).

The interventional treatment possibilities in cardiology increase every year. It is not the purpose of this book to discuss the reasonableness of individual developments or

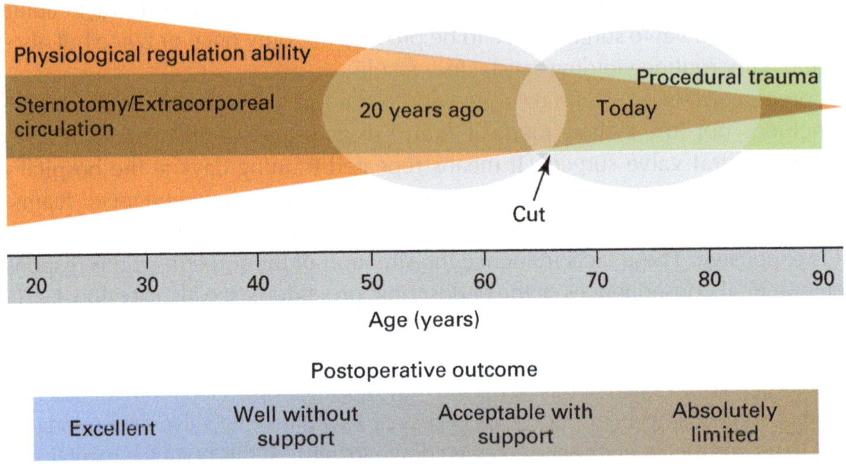

Fig. 1.2: Physiological regulation abilities (red triangle) of many corporeal functions decrease with age. For a given procedural trauma (blue bar) there will be a point when trauma exceeds the regulation ability (cut). After this point more and more support is necessary after heart surgery to achieve acceptable results for patients. In the subgroup of patients older than 80 years, classical surgery is more often unsuccessful because of those limitations.

the quality of individual results. However, what these methods all have in common is that, as a general rule, the organism's stress level is significantly lower during the treatment. Hence, what is decisive for heart surgery is the fact that with every new form of interventional treatment as an alternative to conventional surgery, the pressure grows to question the application of the adequate surgical method in the present form.

An older patient population and changed expectations of younger patients require the development of heart surgical procedures with lower physical stress and better cosmetic results.

Taking into account these cohesions it becomes clear that the introduction of a program of endoscopic mitral valve repair only represents the implementation of more and more changing requirements of heart surgery. Future development leads away from extensive heart surgery to an endoscopic procedure, a procedure that will increasingly be combined with interventional treatment methods. The combination of percutanous transluminal coronary angioplasty (PTCA) and endoscopic valve intervention instead of open and combined surgery is mentioned here as an example.

Hence, the introduction of endoscopic mitral valve surgery is more than just a new method; it has to be understood as a gateway to the future of heart surgery.

1.2.1 Starting conditions for endoscopic mitral valve surgery

Introducing minimally invasive mitral valve surgery into an operating room is normally the idea of the heart surgeon. Often the distinct steps required to develop such a program successfully are underestimated. The course can be outlined in many situations as follows.

The surgeon concentrates on the new technology that he or she has to learn and the instruments that will be needed. The surgeon selects a team from the existing staff to start the new tasks. After discussions with companies that, for example, sell the instruments or by using the team's contacts, an appointment will be scheduled for visiting a hospital that has been using this new technology for a longer time. The surgeon can see that it works and expects that he or she can achieve the same. The decision is made. The program will start.

But what about the necessary budget? Talks are held with the hospital's management. The surgeon definitely wants to work with the latest technology and the administration wants to invest as little money as possible and wants to wait, if move forward at all. In addition the administration normally wants to know what benefit can be expected from the introduction of a new therapy that requires investment. The administration expects facts and numbers that are usually not available to the surgeon.

A compromise will be found, or less official routes are taken. Instruments will be bought and the first patient will be selected. Because a higher number of patients are not expected in the beginning, one set of instruments seems to be enough. From the available equipment, material such as cannulas and sutures will be selected. A few additional materials will be ordered and the first operation starts. This operation will not be a huge success and will take a relatively long time. But all members of the staff are optimistic and further procedures will be carried out. Everything seems to move in the right direction.

But during one of the next procedures complications might occur. After a time-consuming attempt to repair the valve, valve replacement might be necessary. Bleeding might occur after the end of the operation. Sometimes the procedure seems to be very complex and it will turn out relatively expensive, too. After a few more times some members of the team will lose faith in the new procedure and it will be difficult to justify continuation; the technology will disappear from the catalogue of procedures of the center. Management will be glad that it has been conservative with investments to a great extent and that the surgeon's supposed adventure did not yield essential results.

This outlined sequence of events appears drastic. However, this holds true much too often. Why do many clinics fail to introduce endoscopic heart surgery successfully? The answer to this question is relatively simply: The project is ill prepared.

In the end it is neither about the individual abilities and skills of the surgeon(s) nor about the immediate and concrete preparation of a single operation. It is a matter of introducing this procedure in a systematic trial in a clinic because all parties involved are persuaded by reasonableness and the necessity of this procedure (▶Fig. 1.3).

To support the necessary discussions and to clarify the general purpose, some arguments are explained in the following sections.

1.2.2 Patient-related arguments

Prognosis

The prognosis of patients suffering from extreme mitral valve insufficiency depends substantially on the correction of this condition before secondary damage is caused to the heart. Quite a few of those often relatively young patients have none or just a few

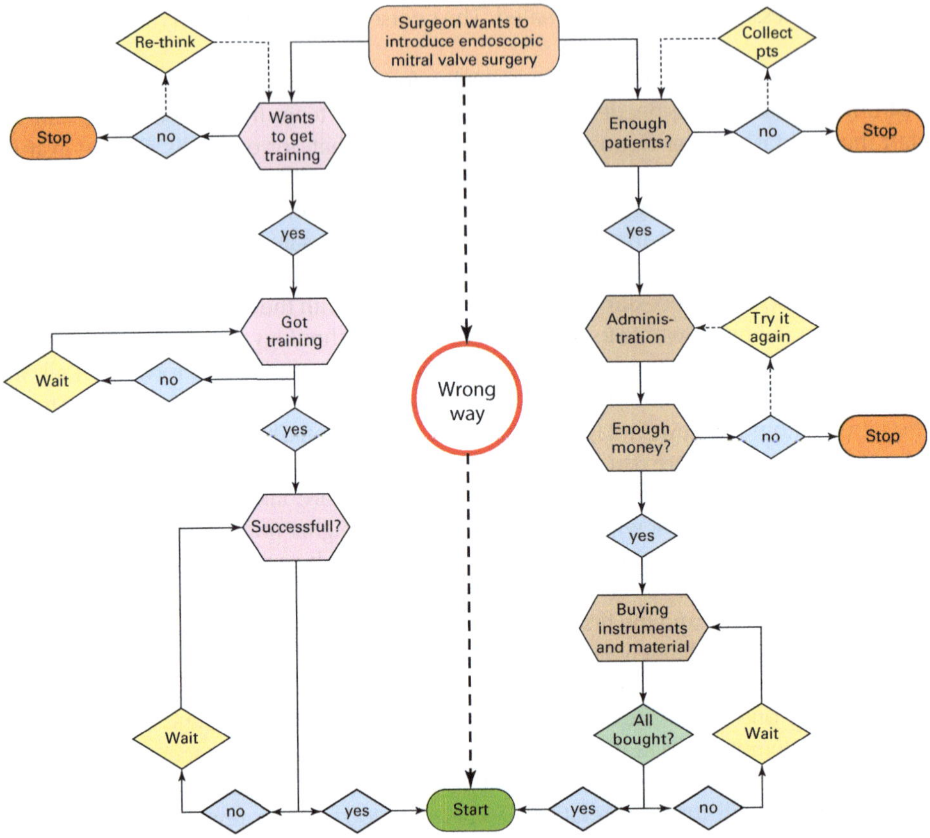

Fig. 1.3: Description of the decision-making process for introducing endoscopic mitral valve surgery. In general there are two parallel processes. On the one hand it is about organizing "material" and financial prerequisites (patients, budget, instruments). On the other hand it is the preparation of the surgeon (and the team) for implementation. If some points cannot be achieved (patients, budget, training) the program should not be implemented. But for any quandary a way out is shown.

complaints at first, although they might suffer from severe valve insufficiency. Some of these patients show beginning dilatation of the left ventricle or beginning pulmonary hypertension.

In order to preserve the chances of success it is necessary to operate on these patients immediately. In the end, the patient's decision to undergo such a procedure is also influenced by imagining a median sternotomy (negatively) or just an endoscopy (positively). In the course of this procedure the assigning cardiologists will expand their consciousness concerning these problems (provided that the results are right). As a result it takes less time to draw up anamnesis before surgery (▶Fig. 1.4).

What are the advantages for the hospital? Patients come earlier, they are younger and healthier at the time of surgery and therefore the potential for complications is minimized. The length of stay and the costs of therapy will be reduced. Things have come full circle.

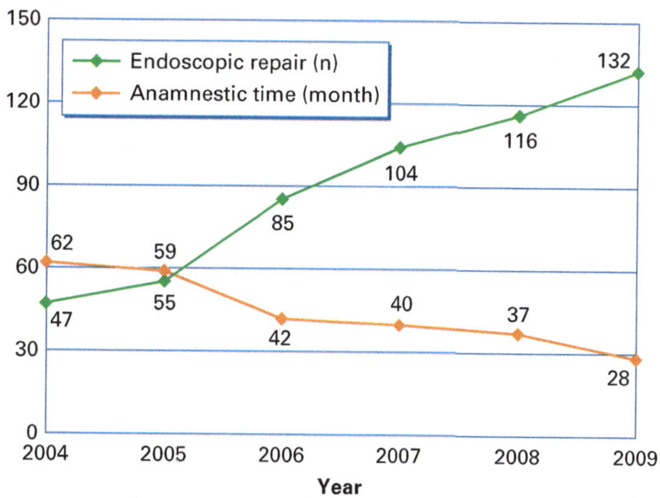

Fig. 1.4: With a growing number of patients per year (green line) and more acceptance of this kind of procedure, the anamnesis duration decreases (orange line). The patients undergo valve repair earlier and show little potential for complications (author's own results).

Need for blood transfusion

The transfusion of blood has two essential aspects: It is expensive and always linked to risks. Hence, all efforts should be made to decrease the necessity of blood transfusions. In contrast to open-heart surgery, the wound surface inside the thoracic cavity and the necessity of preparations with endoscopic interventions are reduced significantly. As a consequence, the bleeding probability and transfusion demand are reduced, as is the case in 30–50% on average requiring blood transfusion after median sternotomy (author's own results).

The decrease of blood transfusions can influence positively the cost structure of endoscopic interventions. Besides the medical advantage of a risk decrease, there is an economic benefit that can be helpful in the discussion with the management of the hospital.

Wound-healing disturbances

Wound-healing disturbances after median sternotomy are one of the mostly dreaded complications after heart surgery. Besides the mostly deleterious results for the patient, they cause an often long-lasting treatment with a high mortality. Associated expenses exceed the proceeds many times over so that the avoidance of this problem is not only to the patient's advantage but also to the clinic's.

Of course, wound-healing disturbances mostly affect patients who have undergone coronary artery bypass grafting. So the potential to do better in mitral valve surgery seems not too high. But the presence of risk factors for developing a wound-healing disturbance depends on regional and cultural specifics. If this incidence is very low the potential to decrease the number of patients with wound-healing problems is naturally low and, hence, not an argument. But if it is not low the improvement of this situation should be a point.

One of the essential reasons for the development of wound-healing disturbances after median sternotomy seems to be the participation of the bone. In particular with diabetics and overweight patients the combination of mechanical burden on the split sternum and the encroachment of the wound healing on a vascular and cellular level are common issues. Nevertheless, avoiding long-lasting and severe wound-healing problems means not only to prevent these in one patient but also, sometimes, to save more money than it takes to start an endoscopic mitral valve program.

The only way to exclude this risk is the avoidance of the sternotomy. The benefits can be found at three different levels: First, the patient benefits because he or she is not subject to sternal wound-healing disturbance risks. Second, the hospital benefits because expenses for the protracted treatment of such wound-healing disturbances will decrease on average. Third, the heart-surgical center benefits because the image of the hospital improves by the decrease of the rate of wound-healing disturbances.

Cosmetic reason

One of the main arguments against minimally invasive mitral valve repair surgery is the insinuation that the procedure is carried out only because of cosmetic reasons.

Can that really be an argument against this intervention? Cosmetic concerns only are certainly insufficient reasons to apply this procedure. But, of course, this concern is also a reason to carry out this procedure. Why should women and men at a younger age live their whole life with a long scar in the middle of their chest after a successful mitral valve repair? These patients are usually healthy and have normal prognoses. Physical intactness belongs to quality of life. Hence, a preserved or only limited cosmetic intactness will contribute substantially to the improvement of the quality of life (▶Fig. 1.5).

The possible medical consequences of sternotomy will be described in the "Wound-healing disturbances" section of Chapter 1.2.2. Nevertheless, median sternotomy also has psychological effects before surgery (decreasing readiness to undergo the procedure) and after surgery (effect of the scar). This is again a matter of the timeliness of this intervention. Help the patient decide on time on such a procedure while distracting his

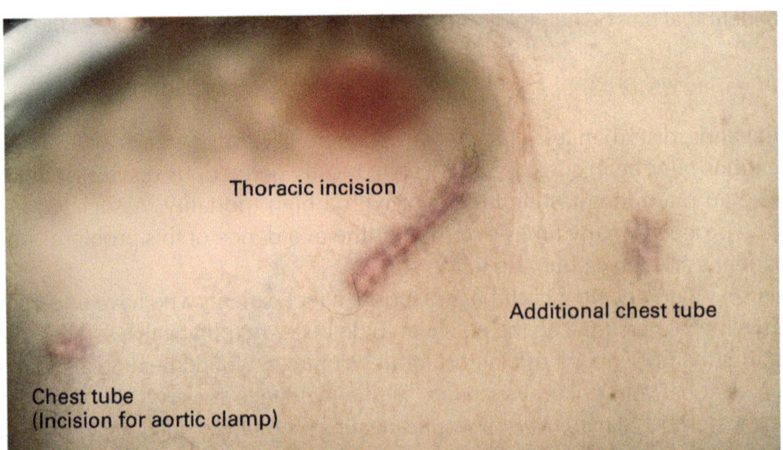

Fig. 1.5: A typical cosmetic result after minimally invasive mitral valve repair in a 52-year-old man, 6 months after procedure.

or her fears of sternotomy consequences and complications. Recommend an endoscopic intervention to the patient.

1.2.3 Hospital-related arguments

Marketing

Whether you work at a private heart center, public hospital, or as a freelance heart surgeon with your own patients, patients and cardiologists base their decision on where such a treatment should take place not only on the external circumstances of the place of treatment but also, above all, on the possibilities offered and, of course, the quality of the results.

Today – in the times of an occasional abundance of capacity for heart surgery on one hand and the economic necessities on the other[1] – competition between hospitals has become normal. There are numerous medical reasons that speak for endoscopic mitral valve repair. Nevertheless, another option is to reach a regionally or nationally unique characteristic, too. Together with the possibility of a certain and often additional number of patients resulting from it, the introduction of such a method becomes very attractive.

At present there is generally no exhaustive supply to carry out interventions on the mitral valve and/or the tricuspid valve as well as the closure of an atrial septal defect in endoscopic technology. From it arises with certain coerciveness that the clinic can reach a competitive advantage if it shows such a supply in its spectrum. Nevertheless, it should be pointed out at this moment that the consideration of a competitive advantage only is no sufficient criterion for the introduction of this procedure. But it is a factor that can help make lasting decisions.

Economic reasons

Endoscopic or minimally invasive surgery pursues the purpose to decrease the traumatic burden on patients. In the case of a minimally invasive procedure, the avoidance of sternotomy remains an essential asset in comparison to open-heart surgery. Nevertheless, this apparently slight difference produces two significant advantages in practice.

In patients without sternotomy the breathing function stays preserved without limitations after the procedure. The complete system of thoracic skeleton and breathing muscles is to a great extent unchanged. The resulting breath mechanics are not impaired by limited movements or fears as very often can be seen after sternotomy. Preexisting lung diseases can be treated substantially better with physiotherapy as well as with active coughing by the patient. As a consequence, the risk of a re-intubation as well as the development of pneumonia decreases dramatically (▶Fig. 1.6).

Another observation showed that apparently the minor manipulation of the heart together with the preservation of the pericardium greatly allows a faster recovery of the heart. Consequently, the stay of the patients in the intensive care unit (ICU) can often be shortened by about one day[2] after a minimally invasive procedure in comparison to patients that undergo sternotomy (author's own data, 2005–2010) (▶Fig. 1.7). The available capacity for intensive-care medicine might be different from hospital to hospital and from country to country. Nevertheless, shortening the stay at the ICU always helps to minimize costs.

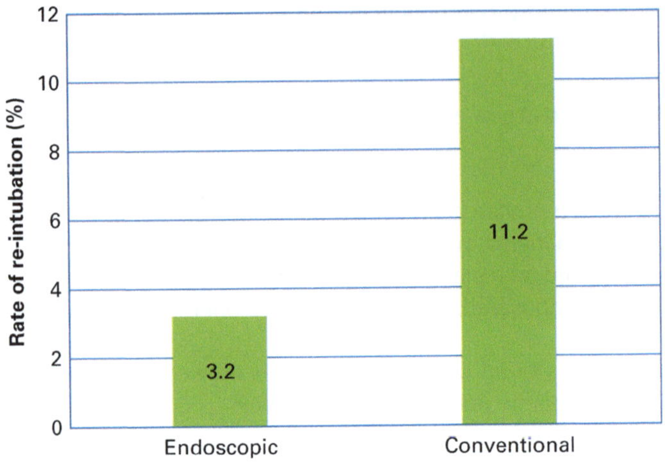

Fig. 1.6: The use of the minimally invasive technology leads to a decrease in the rate of re-intubations (author's own results, 2005–2010).

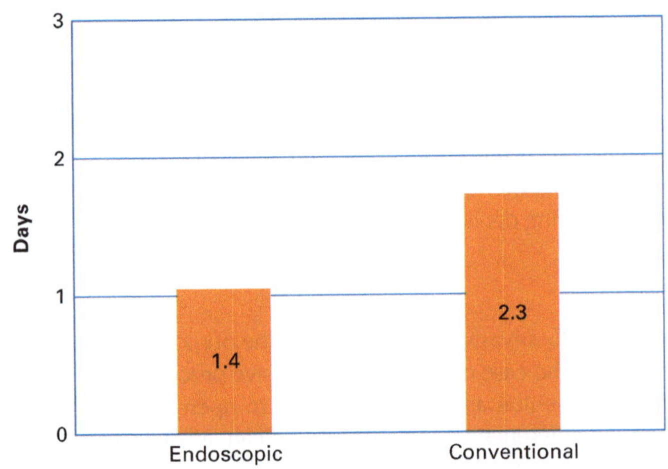

Fig. 1.7: Using minimally invasive technology leads to a shortening of the length of stay in the ICU of about one day (author's own results, 2005–2010).

What is the result? If in a year 50 patients are treated with minimally invasive intervention, about 50 fewer bed days are required. According to the average length of stay at the ICU, between 25 and 50 additional patients can be operated on without increasing staff costs. And personnel costs are always high.

A similar situation is found for the entire stay at the clinic. The minimization of operational trauma leads to a patient's quicker recovery. The result is a similar shortening of the necessary hospital stay duration to possibly one day. Here the same applies as in intensive care: Quicker recovery of a certain number of patients brings additional capacities without additional expenses.

Table 1.1: Expected economic benefits after development of an endoscopic heart surgical program. The numbers here, which are calculated for the health care system in Germany, have to be adapted to country-specific systems.

Criterion	Effects	Benefit	Per 20 cases
Stay at ICU	decreases about one day per patient	+ € 1,100 / patient	+ € 22,000
In-hospital-stay	decreases about one day per patient	+ € 250 / patient	+ € 5,000
Number of operations	increases about one per endoscopic procedure	+ € 2,000 / additional patient	+ € 40,000
Overall			+ € 67,000

The economic benefit can be calculated in a direct and indirect part. The direct part is the decrease of the average treatment costs per patient (decrease of the length of stay at the ICU and at the hospital) as well as in the decrease in the expenditure for the treatment of wound-healing disturbances (avoidance of sternotomy). The height of this direct economic benefit depends, of course, on the respective circumstances of a hospital. Nevertheless, it can be estimated quite accurately on this basis ▶Table 1.1. In particular, the decrease of the length of stay at the ICU opens new possibilities because this is often the bottleneck of heart surgery.

The indirect part is more difficult to calculate. The development of an endoscopic heart surgical program will generally lead after some time to the fact that, with the patients as well as with the collaborating cardiologists' expertise for such interventions, the heart-surgical clinic or the individual surgeon will be committed to this procedure. The reputation of the surgeon increases. It is a frequent psychological mechanism that such an expertise is expanded automatically to other interventions. The result is an increased patient inflow for procedures that have nothing in common with endoscopic heart surgery. In the end, this can lead, together with the additional capacities without additional staff and beds at the intensive care unit, to a higher operation frequency.[3] Subsequently – and this is, for the management of a hospital, quite an essential point – this results in a positive balance.

1.2.4 Patient selection

An essential criterion for the successful implementation of an endoscopic program to reconstruct mitral valves is the careful selection of the first patients. The complexity of the whole intervention is reason enough to keep the necessary steps of the reconstruction of the valve with experienced surgeons as simple as possible. The essential criteria are summarized in ▶Table 1.2.

The basic idea behind a careful patient selection is to specify the conditions for reaching good results at both the beginning and later. These results are marked by a low perioperative risk without mortality and excellent functional results after reconstruction of the valve. It is not important to operate possibly on many and possibly on all patients endoscopically who could have an indication immediately. It is important

Table 1.2: Basic criteria for an adapted patient selection to start an endoscopic mitral valve program. The main idea is to keep the perioperative risk low and make the reconstruction of the valve as simple as possible.

Selection Criterion	Remarks
Age	Between 45 and 70 years; patients younger than 30 years often show a complex valve morphology (Barlow's disease); older patients more often have general health problems
Sex	Males are better candidates than females because of the height of the thorax and the space inside; preparation is easier in males (see Section 4.2)
Weight	Normal weight (or slightly obese, BMI < 30); in obese patients the preparation could be more complicated (see Section 6.2)
LVEF	Quiet normal; decreased LVEF increases the perioperative risk
Valve morphology	Isolated prolapse of P2 that allows a simple quadrangular or triangular resection (see Sections 5.1 and 5.2); avoid isolated prolapses of anterior leaflet segments (see Section 5.5) and isolated ring dilatations with "ventricularized" posterior leaflets (see Section 5.6), no calcification of the annulus
Vessel status	No calcifications of ascending aorta; no stenosis of coronary, femoral, and carotid arteries
Lung function	No severe pulmonary diseases
General	No former cardiac operations (no redo procedures in the beginning)

Note: LVEF = left ventricular ejection fraction.

to convince not only patients and collaborating cardiologists but also the team of the correctness of the new way.

With every patient leaving the clinic in good health and with his or her mitral valve repaired another "advertising media" is generated. The same applies to cardiologists. They will do this again when they have performed surgery on a patient and received a very good result from this endoscopic intervention. A careful selection of the patient also ensures a success for the surgeon. The preservation of the motivation is important because with more complicated patients more difficult situations originate. Here the surgeon must know that he or she can do it (see Section 1.1.3).

But what if not enough "optimum" patients are available or a high number of patients will be sent to the hospital with an indication for a valve replacement? It is incorrect to assume that an endoscopic program cannot be started in such cases. A mitral valve replacement can be carried out via endoscopic access as a reconstruction (see Section 5.7) except for patients with strongly calcified annulus parts. In these cases the conventional technology should be chosen. In the end, the advantages for the surgeon lie in the fact that he or she can learn the general way of the procedure regardless of the number of the patients whose valve should be reconstructed. With every patient this part of the intervention will become safer. And a careful valve replacement always produces a good result. Then, in case of a reconstruction, the way to the valve is already tested and the surgeon can concentrate more on the requirements of the reconstruction, hence the risk is lower, the results are better, and the chances rise to see such patients more often.

1.2.5 Teaching course

Most surgeons have already seen at least once the procedure of endoscopic mitral valve surgery before they decide to include it in their operation spectrum. And it seems relatively clear how the operation has to be performed. Then, the real start seems incomparably more difficult (see also Section 1.2.1). Hence, it makes a lot of sense to undergo a certain learning process. The stubborn pride of an experienced surgeon or too big an ego is out of place.

Teaching course basically comprises two parts. The first part contains, as a general rule, at least one-day sitting in on lectures in a center that is familiar with the procedure. The direct contact with a surgeon experienced in endoscopic surgery, the immediate participation in the operating theater, and the possibility to discuss all steps of the operation directly allow a learning process that creates many conditions for a successful start in the operating room. A second sitting-in on lectures has proven sensible where an anesthetist and the involved nursing staff should take part.

The second part should take place in the operating theater of the surgeon who wants to start with this program. A surgeon experienced in endoscopic procedures takes part actively in the procedures. Ideally, this part should last for at least two days with at least four cases in total. The first operation should be carried out by a guest surgeon to demonstrate an ideal execution of such an intervention to all involved team members. Then, all other operations should be carried out by the surgeon who would like to start with the program under the active support of the guest surgeon.

The last step is the continuation of the program on one's own initiative. Here it is particularly important not to let too much time pass between training and the following procedures. Furthermore, close contact with the "teaching" surgeon and the idea of a Web-based sampling of video sequences for typical situations may help.

1.2.6 Starter kit for endoscopic mitral valve surgery

In discussions with the management of a hospital, personal engagement and persuasiveness always play a role. However, the conviction of a surgeon of the necessity of the introduction of an operation method is a relatively unspecific criterion for the management, so this concern may also be medically plausible.

A clear calculation of what such a plan will cost to be successful is better and more purposeful. Here, the minimum number of operations also plays a role that should be subdivided in order to reach a certain training effect. And, of course, one should also think about what positive economic effects are to be expected (see Section 1.2.3, Economic reasons). ▶Table 1.3 shows the most important figures of the primary expenditure.

The biggest part of the expenses linked to the introduction of an endoscopic operation program are overheads for instruments and the optical system. These amount in this calculation add up to approximately € 100,000. However, this amount can be less if an optical system is already available (see also Section 4.4). It becomes clear in the calculation of economic benefit and primary expenses that with a number of

Table 1.3: Primary costs for starting an endoscopic program.

Issue	Costs per Unit	Overall Costs[1]
Instruments[2]	€30,000	€60,000
Cannulas (ven + art)[3]	€350	€7,000
Sutures 2	€200	€6,000
Soft tissue retractor 2	€200	€6,000
Teaching session[4]	€5,000	€15,000
Videoscopic system[5]	€30,000	€30,000
Camera[6]	€3,000	€6,000
Overall		€130,000

[1]Costs for 20 patients. [2]Two sets. [3]Costs per operation. [4]3 x 2 days. [5]If not already available. [6]One with 30° view; one with 0° view.

20 patients, the biggest part of the primary investment can be compensated. And after 40 patients the primary expenditure has already been worthwhile. Only the current expenditure per operation remains.[4]

However, this arrangement should also prove that it makes no sense to renounce qualitatively adequate and sufficient equipment. Indeed, the acquisition of only one instrument set seems nominal enough to operate on the well-selected isolated cases at the beginning of the program. Nevertheless, in relation to the conditions of real life the second set (or at least the most important parts) should be acquired at the same time. The failure of one or several instruments (mechanical dysfunction, loss of sterility by inadvertent dropping on the floor, or other reasons) can hinder the execution of the operation considerably or make it quite impossible (e.g. Knot pusher). The same applies to the necessity of a rethoracotomy. The reopening of the right-sided incision is no problem; nevertheless, it could become difficult to stop an actually slight bleeding with classical instruments by this access.

1.2.7 Overview

As an overview about the arguments and benefits, the next graphic shows the main facts for all members involved in developing an endoscopic mitral valve repair program (▶Fig. 1.8). Some of these arguments and benefits depend on the specific situation of the hospital and the interests of the hospital's owner. Others depend on the personal situation of the surgeon and the country where he or she works. But all of these will help to achieve the prerequisites for the successful introduction of a program for endoscopic mitral valve surgery.

Patient	• Repair before secondary damages of the heart occurs • Lower perioperative risk • Faster recovery • No sternotomy/no scare • No risk of wound-healing disturbances
Surgeon	• Enlargement of procedural options • More options in the competition between hospitals • Improves skills and results • Requires more patients • Moves into the future of heart surgery
Administration	• Improves the cost/earnings relation of the hospital • Makes the hospital fit for competition with other hospitals • Get payed back the investment multiple • Improves the use of OR/ICU capacity
Cardiologist	• Get additional options for his or her patients • Is motivated to send the patients early enough for mitral valve repair • Improves his or her practice in collaboration with the surgeon

Fig. 1.8: Conclusion of advantages and benefits for all parties involved when an endoscopic program for mitral valve surgery is started.

Notes

1. This might be specific for industrialized countries, but marketing is necessary everywhere.
2. Some hospitals already have fast-track protocol where most patients typically stay only one day in the ICU.
3. Capacity is not the limited factor everywhere. However, a paid bed should be used in maximum.
4. The calculation of reimbursement is based on the German health care system with a payment that follows the so-called diagnose related groups system (DRG 2010). For other systems or private hospitals, the numbers have to be adapted.

2 Anesthesiology and pain management

2.1 Intubation and ventilation

In endoscopic mitral valve surgery under the conditions of a retrograde perfusion and a broken ventilation it is necessary to ensure that the oxygen supply of the brain is guaranteed. For control of this situation the surgeon, the anesthetist, and the perfusionist have to understand the mechanisms if a physiological antegrade and an artificial retrograde perfusion operate at the same time.

Especially after starting the extracorporeal circulation at the beginning of the operation and at the time after closing the atrium and controlling the result with the transesophageal echocardiogram (TEE), we find a sufficient antegrade perfusion because of the filling of the heart. Dependent on the perfusion pressure and the ejected volume of the left ventricle and persistent retrograde perfusion, a zone of mixed blood consisting out of oxygenated and nonoxygenated blood results if there is no ventilation (for details see Section 6.1).

Defining the location of the so-called mixed zone is very difficult and therefore represents a danger for having a seemingly efficient perfusion of the supraaortic vessels but in reality there is a lack of cerebral oxygenation because the cerebral perfusion results from an antegrade cardiac output.

> To be sure at any time of a sufficient cerebral oxygen supply during retrograde perfusion it should be a standard technique to use a double lumen tube with isolated left lung ventilation at the beginning and the end of the operation.

Because of this context, we always perform a single lung ventilation (of the left lung, of course) at the beginning and the end of the operation. That means that we start with the ECG with continuous left lung ventilation until the heart is empty, so the antegrade output is zero. Now you can be absolutely sure that retrograde perfusion will reach the supraaortic vessels with safe cerebral oxygenation. The same procedure is carried out at the end of the operation after declamping the aorta and starting the antegrade output of the heart. Here we start with left lung ventilation when the oxygen saturation of the blood (of course measured at the right hand) is lower than 90%.

A prerequisite for such a process is to have a side-separated intubation (▶Fig. 2.1). The different techniques to bring a double lumen tube in the right position are well described in anaesthesiological textbooks.

2.2 Pain management

One of the arguments against endoscopic or minimally invasive mitral valve surgery is the assertion that patients operated on in such a manner have more and long-lasting postoperative pain than patients after sternotomy.

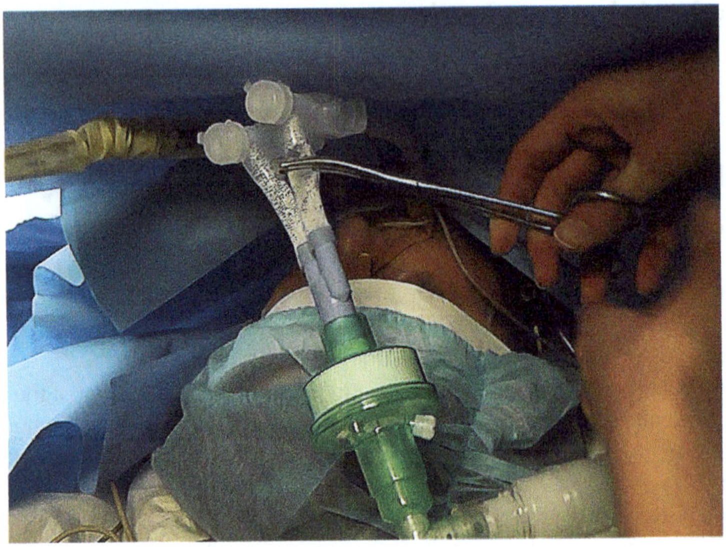

Fig. 2.1: Correctly placed double lumen tube allows single left lung ventilation at the beginning and the end of the operation.

That is not generally true, but it is right that the manipulation of the ribs sometimes (especially in older patients) can lead to pain similar to that experienced after a rib contusion. The result is a lower respiratory excursion with a flatter inspiration and a higher risk to develop pneumonia following surgery.

To prevent these problems it is necessary to start sufficient pain management intraoperatively. There are two different ways to work on it – anaesthesiological pain management with drugs in a sufficient dose and surgical opportunities.

Efficient pain management is more important for the early postoperative period than for a longer time. It combines surgical methods with intercostal injections at the end of the operation and overlapping intravenous and/or subcutaneous medication for the first days following surgery.

The first step to prevent postoperative pain is to make a small incision between the ribs and to avoid spreading the ribs too wide. The use of the videoscopic technique helps to reduce that risk very effectively (see also Section 4.4). Experience shows that an intercostal injection of 10 ml Ropivacain® at each wound pole before closing the wound leads to a pain-free situation after the patient awakes (▶Fig. 2.2). The effect generally lasts from 4 to 6 hours. Overlapping to that mechanism, sufficient pain medication has to be administered after extubation of the patient for one to two days or even longer if the patient feels pain for a longer time.

In very rare cases (<0.05%) a really long-lasting pain on the right thoracic side can disturb the quality of life of the affected patients. Here a potentially different reason must be considered for this problem, discussed, and any orthopedic reason must be excluded (e.g. a chronic pain situation of the vertebral column). If all other reasons were excluded

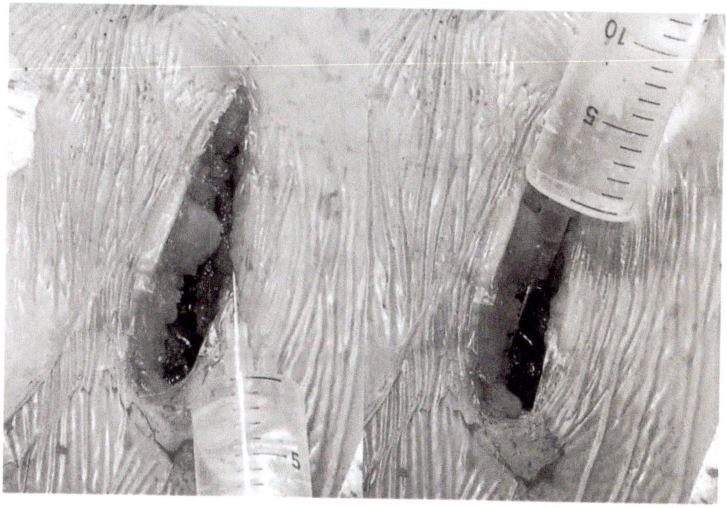

Fig. 2.2: Injection of Ropivacain® into the intercostal space at both wound poles for preventing postoperative pain.

a chronic pain therapy with repeat intercostal injections of anesthetics should be performed. In our experience most of these patients will be pain free after a maximum of 12–24 months.

3 Technical prerequisites

3.1 Cannulas and extracorporeal circulation

3.1.1 Arterial cannulas (retrograde perfusion)

The cannulas for arterial retrograde perfusion that are on the market all seem to have the same structure. The complete set includes a small cannula for aspiration of the femoral artery, a guidewire, some dilators, the introducer, and the cannula itself (▶Fig. 3.1). The size depends on the necessary perfusion volume and the diameter of the femoral artery and reaches from 16 F or 18 F (in few cases) over 19 F to 20 F (in most cases) to 23 F to 24 F for larger patients.

The main differences between some models result from the thickness of the cannula wall (the difference between the inner and the outer diameter), the length of the introducer, which comes out of the tip of the cannula, and the shape of the transition area between the introducer and the cannula.

For a given outer diameter (the size in French) the inner diameter is decisive for the flow characteristics and, in the end, the flow resistance of the cannula (▶Fig. 3.2). That means that under unfavorable conditions there is a high perfusion resistance without the presence of a technical error. It seems to be important for each surgeon who wants to start endoscopic mitral valve surgery that he or she tries different arterial cannulas under different conditions to find the best setting for the patient.

The length of the introducer at the outside of the tip of the cannula is important for the risk estimation for vessel perforation during the introduction of the cannula. If the patient has distinctive tortuous arteries and/or some calcifications in the more proximal parts of the femoral or iliac artery it is very important to control the position of the tip of

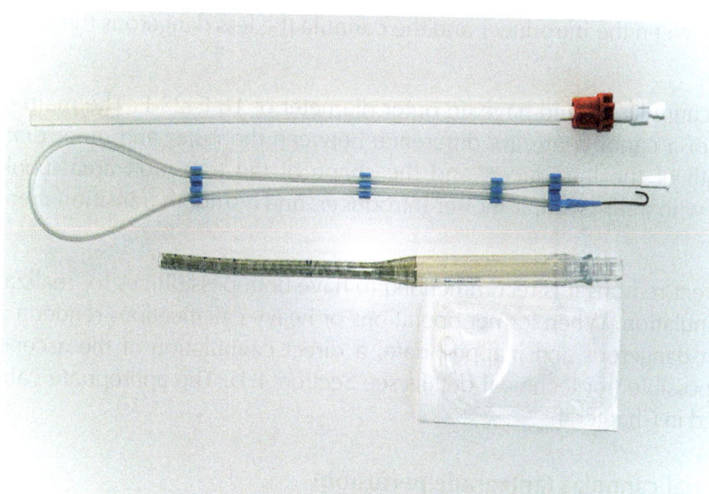

Fig. 3.1: A complete set of an arterial cannula. It includes a needle for aspiration, the guidewire, an introducer, and the cannula itself.

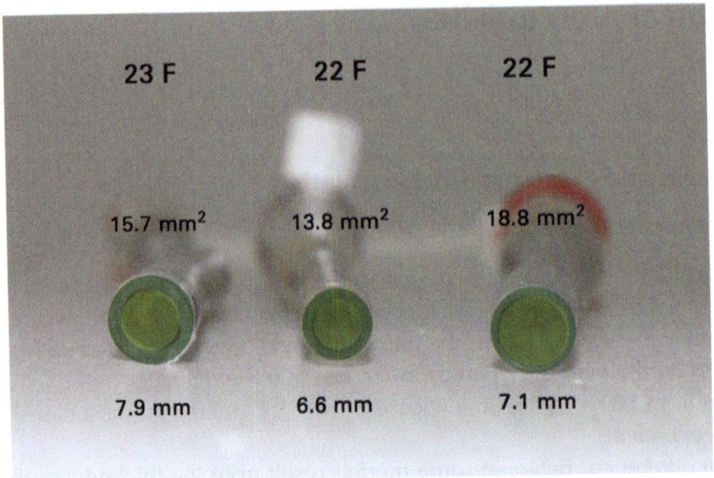

Fig. 3.2: Different outer and inner diameters of different cannula models. Flow resistance will be influenced by these characteristics.

the cannula exactly. That means, if it is necessary to put in a longer part of the introducer at first, followed by the cannula over a longer distance, the tip of the introducer can damage the vessel or rupture a plaque before the cannula itself has safely been positioned. This bad situation must be avoided, and the main method is to use a shorter introducer system (▶Fig. 3.3).

Another main point is the transition area between the introducer and the tip of the cannula. Most cannulas have a conical tip, the base of which has a diameter that is a bit wider than the diameter of the introducer (▶Fig. 3.4). This transition area is distinctive for a safe introduction of the cannula, especially in those cases where the inner diameter of the vessel is only a bit larger than the outer diameter of the cannula, or where a certain degree of calcification avoids dilating the vessel. The smother the transition between the introducer and the cannula the less dangerous the introduction.

> Arterial cannulas should have an outer diameter of 16 F–23 F. The main characteristics of a cannula are the difference between the outer and inner diameters, the length of the introducer, and the shape of the transition area. Look for a cannula with a thin wall, a shorter introducer, and a smooth transition area.

For different reasons it is recommended to have both possibilities for realization of an arterial cannulation. When former operations or heavy calcifications render a peripheral cannulation dangerous and inappropriate, a direct cannulation of the ascending aorta should be possible (for technical details see Section 4.1). The appropriate cannulas will be described in Chapter 4.

3.1.2 Arterial cannulas (antegrade perfusion)

Either for a standard technique or as an alternative procedure for patients with peripheral artery disease or small vessels, a direct cannulation of the ascending aorta can help

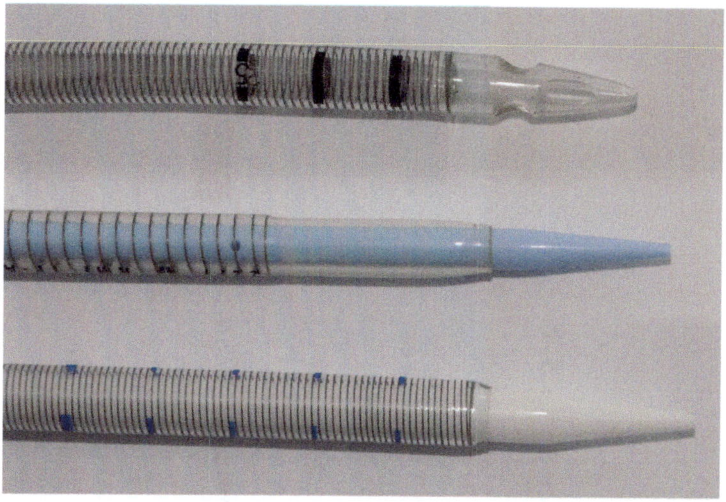

Fig. 3.3: A comparison of introducers in different types of arterial cannulas. The shorter the introducer the smaller the probability of a vessel injury.

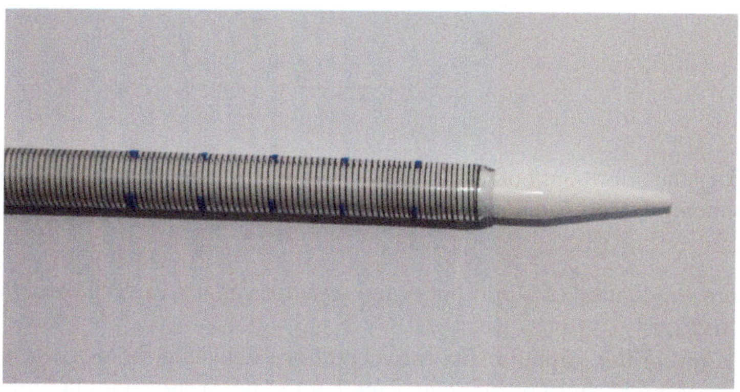

Fig. 3.4: Detailed figure of a transition area between the introducer and the cannula itself. The smoother the transition the lower the probability of vessel damage.

to realize the endoscopic access. For that procedure a special cannula can be used that allows traversing the thoracic wall or directly through the right-sided incision (for details see Section 4.1). This cannula is either similar to the cannulas being used in open-heart surgery (▶Fig. 3.5) or a model with a shorter tip. The main point is to be sure that the intraaortic part is not too long to prevent damage to the opposite aortic wall. Otherwise the same rules apply as for aortic cannulation in open-heart surgery.

3.1.3 Venous cannulas

One of the main prerequisites for undisturbed working on the valve is to evacuate the blood out of the heart reliably and safely while extracorporeal circulation (ECC) is running. One technique to achieve this is to use two cannulas – one in the femoral and one in the jugular vein. Today there is a model on the market that allows the

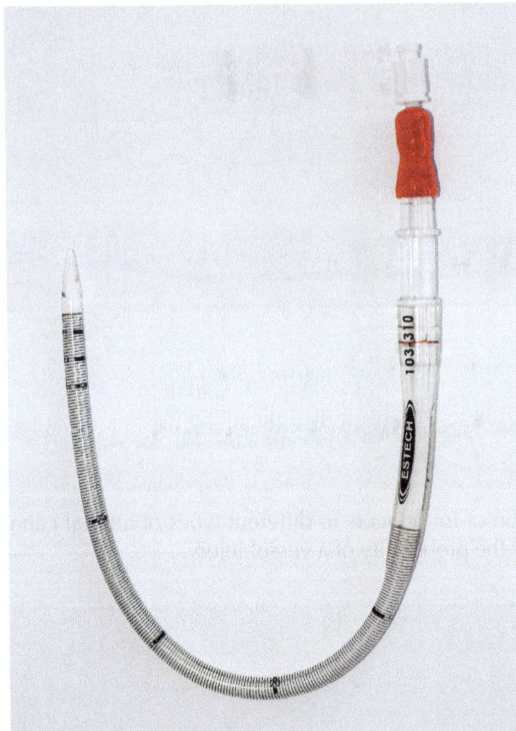

Fig. 3.5: A cannula for transthoracic direct cannulation of ascending aorta or through the mini-thoracotomy (Estech, San Ramon, CA, USA).

simultaneous evacuation of blood out of the superior vena cava (SVC) and the inferior vena cava (IVC).

The structure of this cannula shows two portions with inlet holes over a length of about 10 cm. One of these portions is placed at the tip of the cannula and one more distal in a distance of about 12 cm (▶Fig. 3.6). After exact positioning of the cannula, the tip is placed in the SVC, the distal portion with inlet holes is placed in the IVC, and the part without holes is placed in the right atrium.

Besides the comfortable evacuation of blood, this structure allows additional procedures in the right atrium (tricuspid repair, closure of atrial septal defect type II (ASD) without any additional cannula (for details see Sections 7.3 and 7.4).

For handling of venous cannulas it is important to be able to use both femoral veins. Sometimes it is difficult to introduce the cannula to the right atrium without any resistance in the abdominal part. This can be found in patients with venous thrombosis, former abdominal operations, and traumatic damage to the venous system at one side. If it is necessary to use the other (the left) side, the anatomical way of the vein will cross to the right side in the lower abdominal part. This means that the cannula has to be highly flexible without a loss of functionality. In comparison to different models of venous cannulas, a clear difference in the stiffness or even in the flexibility can be shown (▶Fig. 3.7).

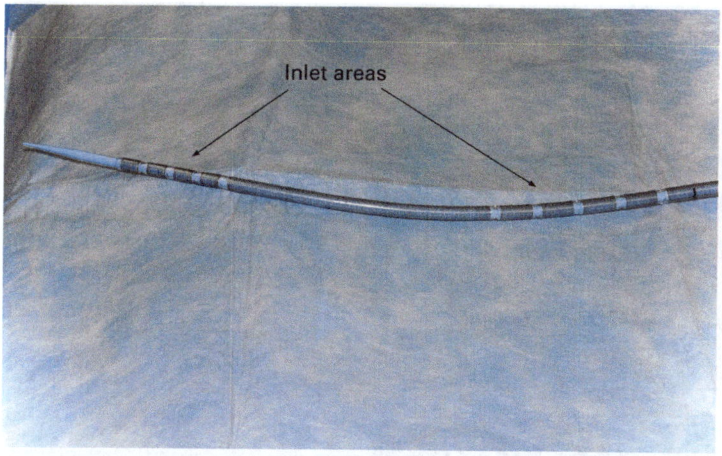

Fig. 3.6: Venous cannula with two areas of inlet holes. This guarantees an excellent volume evacuation and allows procedures in the right atrium without any additional cannula (Estech, San Ramon, CA, USA, 2009).

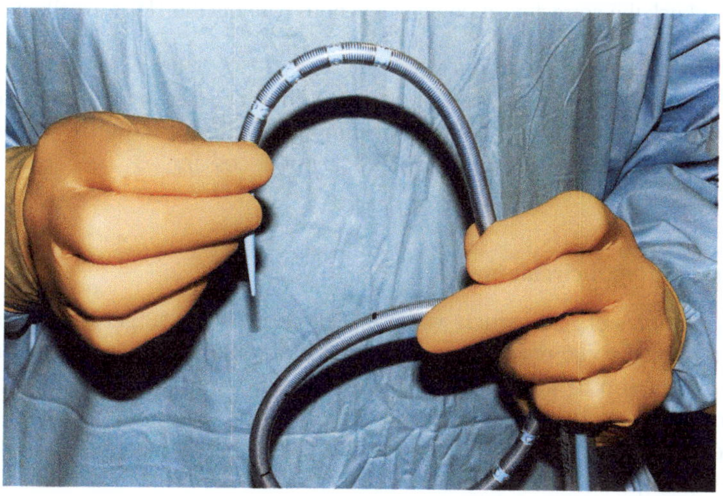

Fig. 3.7: High flexibility allows a successful crossing of the abdominal part of veins (Estech, San Ramon, CA, USA, 2009).

In all patients the diameter of the femoral vein is large enough to use a cannula that allows an effective evacuation of blood. Depending on the body surface of the patient and on the necessary blood flow, a cannula of 20–25 F should be used.

The transition between the introducer system and the venous cannula itself is especially important in the case of a percutaneous implantation of the cannula. Together with a direct arterial cannulation of the ascending aorta this technique allows avoiding an incision of the femoral vessels (for technical details see Section 4.1).

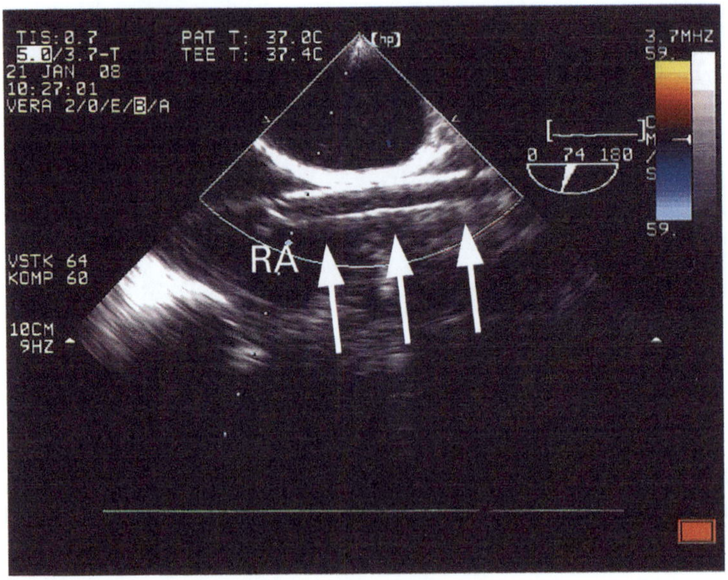

Fig. 3.8: To check the correct positioning of a venous cannula the TEE is excellent to use.

Modern venous cannulas have two portions with inlet holes and a high flexibility. It allows both procedures in the right atrium and in the left atrium. The diameter should be at least 20 F, but more than 24 F is not necessary.

3.1.4 Extracorporeal circulation

The main principles of ECC, which we know from open-heart surgery, are also completely valid for endoscopic procedures. The main difference is the use of venous suction for blood evacuation to support a complete unloading of the heart. This should be a routine procedure to reach a stable and reproducible setting for endoscopic procedures. Adequate evacuation of the heart requires a TEE-assisted optimal positioning of the cannula (▶Fig. 3.8).

There is only one additional rule for ECC in endoscopic procedures – the routine suction on the venous line. All other rules orientate toward the rules of ECC in open-heart surgery.

3.2 Accessories

3.2.1 Soft-tissue retractor

One of the main additional technical tools is the so-called soft-tissue retractor, a device that allows pulling back the soft tissue around the main incision at the right thoracic side. Different models can be found on the market but the construction principle is the same. It contains a ring in different sizes that should be brought into the inner side of the thoracic wall and some lips (or an outer ring) of an elastic tissue with a surface to be glued at the outside. The inner ring works as fixation and the elastic lips allow pulling back the tissue around the incision and fixing it with the surface to be glued (▶Figs. 3.9 and 3.10).

> The optimal soft-tissue retractor contains a relatively small inner ring with wider lips. For practical use, a retractor without any gap between the lips after fixation will be best.

In practical use the main differences result from the wideness of the lips. If there is a smaller wideness after fixation of the tissue some gaps between the lips can result. As a consequence, tissue (especially fatty tissue) can be in the way into the thoracic cavity and so the use of the knot pusher can be aggravated because small tissue parts are brought in. It is toilsome to fetch back these small parts; it takes time and it is not harmless. The best way to prevent this situation is through the use of a soft-tissue retractor with wider lips.

3.2.2 Arms for videoscopic camera and atrial retractor

Of course there are different stabilizers in use for the videoscopic camera and the atrial hook. But it seems to be advantageous to choose a stabilizer that can work with a high stability and an easy handling. This means that someone could use any complex

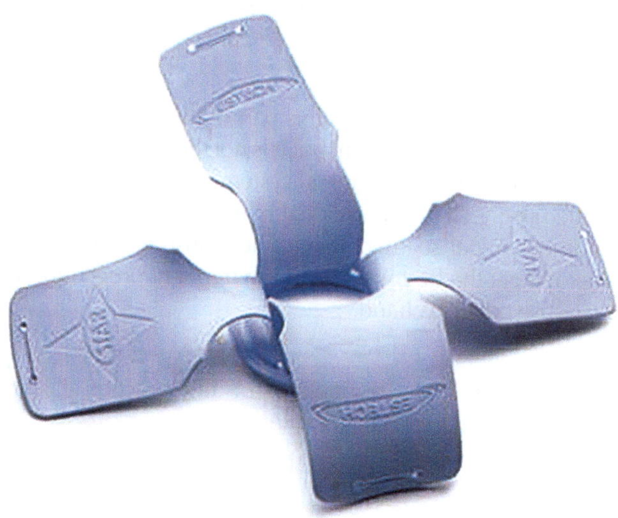

Fig. 3.9: Typical example of a soft-tissue retractor. The ring will be placed inside the thorax and the wide lips allow holding back the soft tissue around the mini-thoracotomy (Estech, San Ramon, CA, USA, 2009).

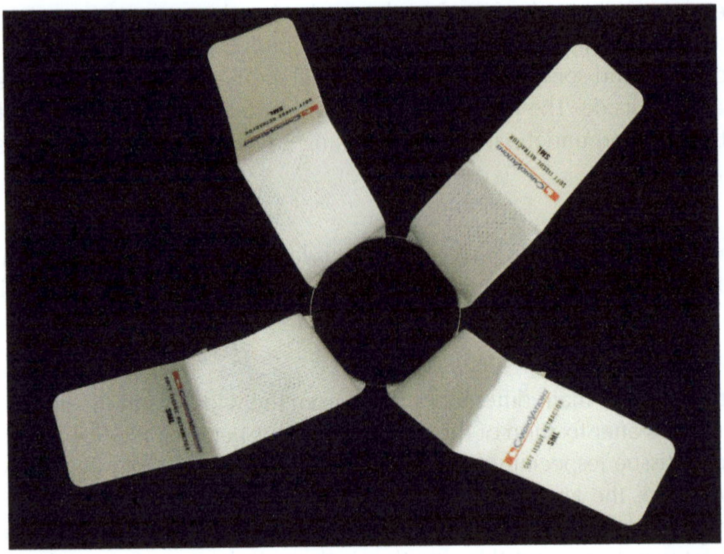

Fig. 3.10: Another example for a soft-tissue retractor. The smaller diameter of the ring allows its use for smaller incisions (Edwards Lifesciences, Irvine, CA, USA, 2009).

system, such as a high-end technique with voice control and/or pneumatic drive, but in the end there is only one reason to use a system for the camera or the hook: to bring and to keep it in a stable position.

The arms for keeping the videoscopic camera and the atrial retractor should be stable, easy to handle, and not too complex. One-hand handling should be preferred.

On the other side it should be clear that this part of the technical equipment is absolutely important for an easygoing operation, but it is not the primary part of the operation.

Because of that, an arm with a mechanical system for fixation of the camera and the hook is recommended (▶Fig. 3.11). In an ideal manufacturing, it is possible to fix or to let off the different mechanical segments with one adjusting screw. Since a small correction of the camera to get the best view will be a frequent procedure during surgery it is very practicable to use only one hand.

Additional tools can help make some steps of an operation easier, especially when the anatomical situation is unfavorable.

3.3 Instruments

Despite the similarity of the instruments for endoscopic cardiac surgery available today there are important differences. In principle it seems to be more reasonable to buy

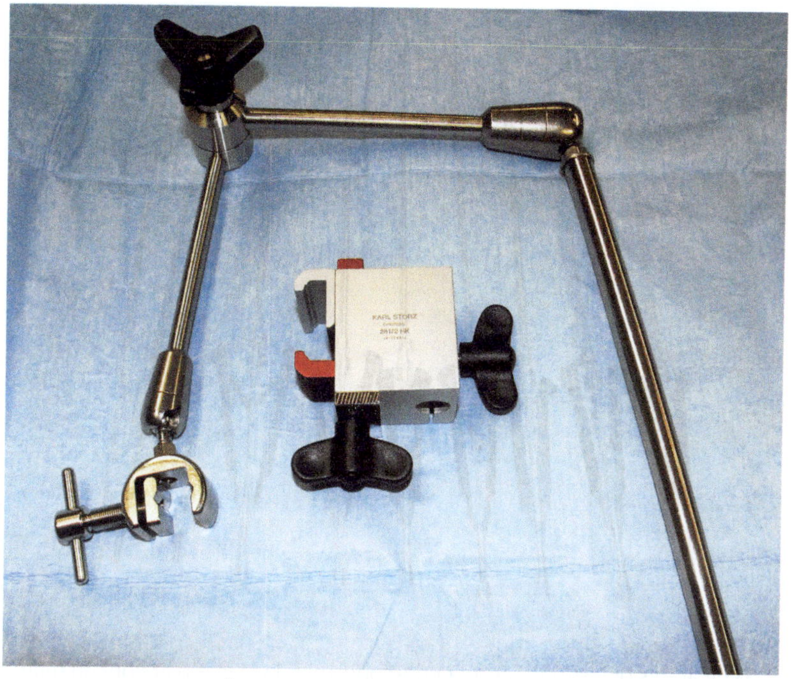

Fig. 3.11: Typical arms for stabilization of scope and atrial hook. The opportunity for central fixation with one adjusting screw allows the device to be worked with only one hand during surgery (Storz, Tuttlingen, Germany).

longer instruments than shorter ones. The mechanical stability and the quality of the areas of the forceps and needle holders, which are intended to hold the tissue and the needles, are important selection criteria (▶Fig. 3.12).

> The quality of the instruments depends on the mechanical stability and the quality of the end parts. The manual force needed to open and close the instruments and to hold the tissue and the needles plays an especially important role.

Meanwhile, different reconstructive techniques were developed. Depending on the situation and the technique used, instruments in different strengths and shapes will be needed (▶Fig. 3.13). Manufacturers of endoscopic instruments definitely take these entitlements into account. The overall number of instruments orientates by the number of operations per day, the rolling period of the sterilization department, and the compliance with redo operations according to a rethoracotomy for the therapy of a possibly postoperative complication. It has to be respected that in the concrete situation of a failure of a specific instrument (e.g. the knot pusher or a fine forceps), either the success of the reconstruction or the endoscopic procedure in principle can be endangered.

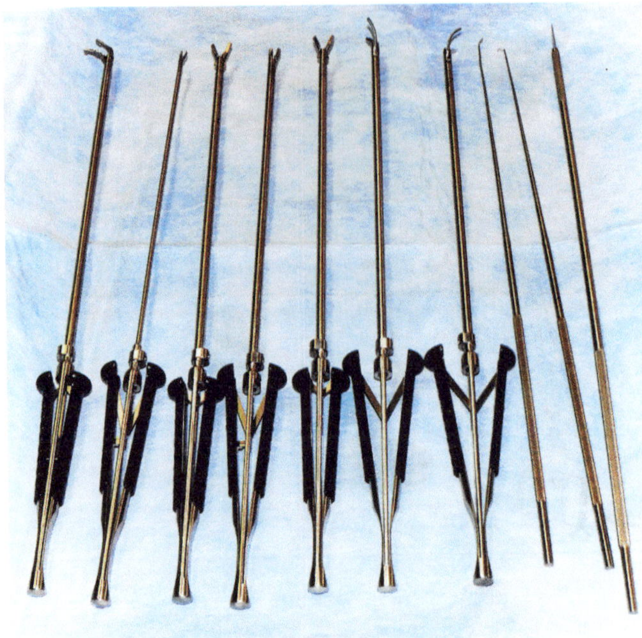

Fig. 3.12: Typical sets of instruments for endoscopic mitral valve repair contain different scissors and forceps, nerve hooks, and a long knife handle (Estech, San Ramon, CA, USA, 2009).

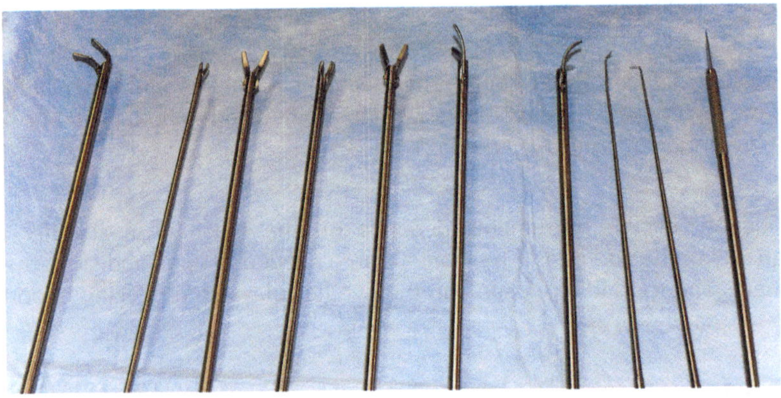

Fig. 3.13: Detailed figure of the special formed tips of the instruments. Forceps and scissors are different in shape and size (Estech, San Ramon, CA, USA, 2009).

It is highly recommended that two sets of instruments are available. In all cases that result from intraoperative nonsterility, rethoracotomy, technical problems with an instrument, or additional cases, the immediate need for additional instruments may occur.

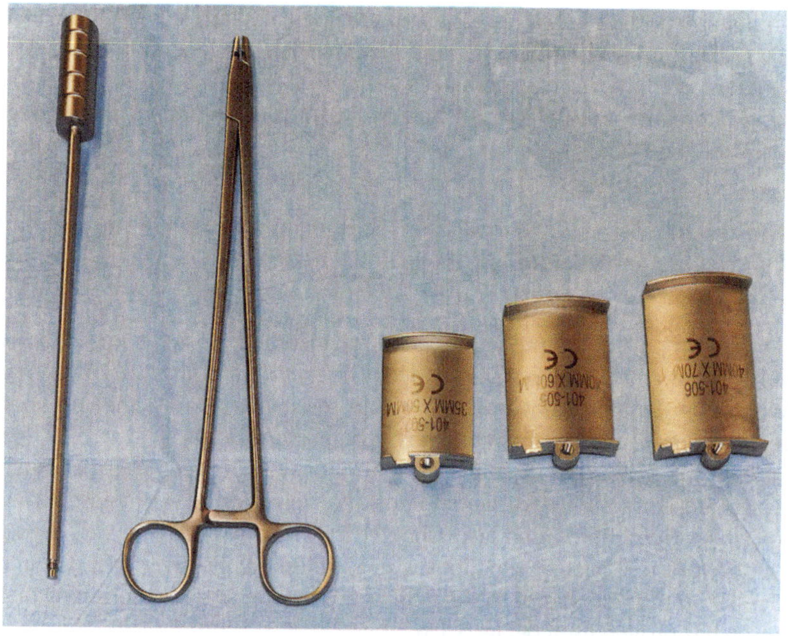

Fig. 3.14: Complete set of atrial hooks. The blades are different in size and will be selected to fit the atrial size.

3.3.1 Atrial hook

The atrial hook is one of the most important and helpful devices of an endoscopic setting. It is made up of a bar in different lengths with a thread at the end and atrial blades in different sizes (▶Fig. 3.14). The construction allows bringing in the bar to the thoracic cavity through an intercostal space. An atrial blade that is fitted to the atrial size is brought into the left atrium and bar and blade will be screwed together.

After screwing together bar and blade, the hook is complete and pulling back the bar the roof of the left atrium will be lifted up for comfortable access to the valve. When the correct position is reached the bar will be connected with the stabilization arm and will be fixed.

The same construction can be used for tricuspid repair, for closure of a small atrial septum defect from the left atrium, and for excision of a tumor out of the left atrium. In these cases a smaller and shorter blade will be advantageous.

3.4 Sutures

The kinds of sutures that are used for endoscopic mitral valve surgery are quite the same as those used for open-heart surgery. In the end the technique for valve repair does not differ in the kind of access. One has to distinguish between sutures for the general part of the operation, such as the cannulation, the opening, and the closure of the thoracic cavity and the left atrium, and the special need for the valve repair.

For all general parts it is not necessary to use special sutures. Here the well-known Prolene® sutures are absolutely sufficient. Size and length depend on the preferences of the surgeon. We have good experiences with a 5–0 Prolene® suture with a one-third needle for sutures of femoral vessels and a 3–0 or 4–0 suture for cardioplegia and closure of the left atrium.

> For the general parts of the operation no special sutures are necessary. The well-known Prolene® sutures are the material of choice.

For the special part of the procedure – the repair of the valve – some additional sutures with special characteristics are needed. The mitral valve is a very dynamic structure. As well as dynamic movement, a stable resistance against the left ventricular pressure during myocardial contraction has to be preserved.

That means the need for a more elastic suture for working on the leaflets such as for closure of a gap, for suturing the leaflet parts after resection of a prolapse, or even the shortening of native chords (see also Chapter 5). We always use a very smooth and elastic suture for these special situations (e.g. Cardionyl®, Peters, Paris). For annuloraphy, a 3–0 suture; for closure of the leaflets, a 4–0 suture; and for shortening of chords, a 5–0 suture has proved itself (▶Fig. 3.15).

On the other side, a more stable suture with lower elasticity is necessary for implantation of neochords. Here the focus has to be directed to a defined length that does not alter during the contraction cycle. Because these sutures are always in blood contact they have to be very smooth and anti-thrombotic. From our experience a 5–0 Gore Tex® suture with a length of 90 cm and one-third needle showed the best results. For details of use see also Chapter 5.

The kind of suture for implantation of an artificial ring depends on the kind of ring. More flexible rings need a more flexible and smooth material for a running suture. The classic rigid rings have to be fixed with sutures with a woven surface, enough length for

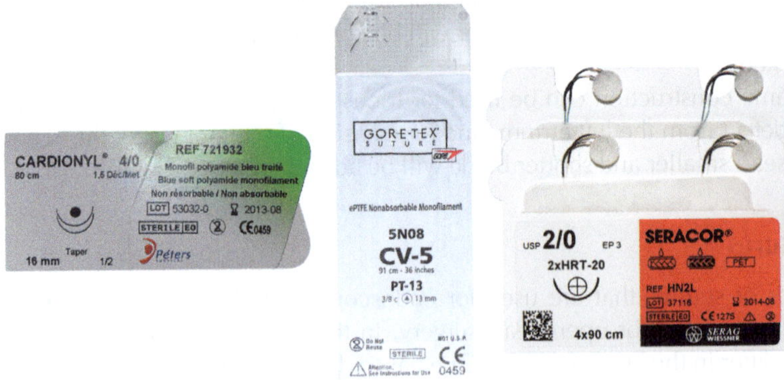

Fig. 3.15: Typical examples of commonly used sutures in mitral valve repair (left: Cardionyl®, Peters, Paris, French; middle: Gore Tex®, Santec Medicalprodukte, Großwallstadt, Germany; right: Valve sutures [Seracor®; Serag Wiessner, Naila, Germany]).

knotting, and good gliding features. All these attributes were combined in the 90 cm long 3–0 suture from Serag Wiessner, Germany (see also Section 5.6).

Special parts of the operation need special sutures. For repair of the leaflets, the implantation of neochords, and the implantation of artificial rings, different sutures should be chosen.

4 Preparations

4.1 Arterial and venous cannulation

One standard for arterial and venous cannulation is to bring in the cannulas into the femoral vessels. There are two different ways to do that: the first is to prepare the vessels with a small cutaneous incision and perform a cannulation directly, the second is to use a transcutaneous technique.

4.1.1 Femoral vessel cannulation after preparation

The first step is the cutaneous incision, which should be made longitudinally and parallel to the anatomical course of the vessels. It is important to make the incision a bit lateral to the femoral artery (▶Fig. 4.1). Then the preparation should go deeper until the level of the vessels is reached, at which point there is a good opportunity to prepare more in the direction of the vessels (i.e., more to the medial). That helps to be sure that there is no harm of lymphatic nodes, which are often found in the region directly above the vessels, and helps avoid the opportunity of postoperative lymphatic fistulas.

To get an opportunity to clamp the vessels in cases of complications with bleeding (i.e., rupture of a suture after removing the cannulas), it is necessary to prepare the vessels so that there is enough space to bring in a clamp (▶Fig. 4.2). Then a circular suture marks the region where the cannulas should be brought in. These sutures are used for closing the holes in the vessels after removing the cannulas at the end of ECC (▶Fig. 4.3).

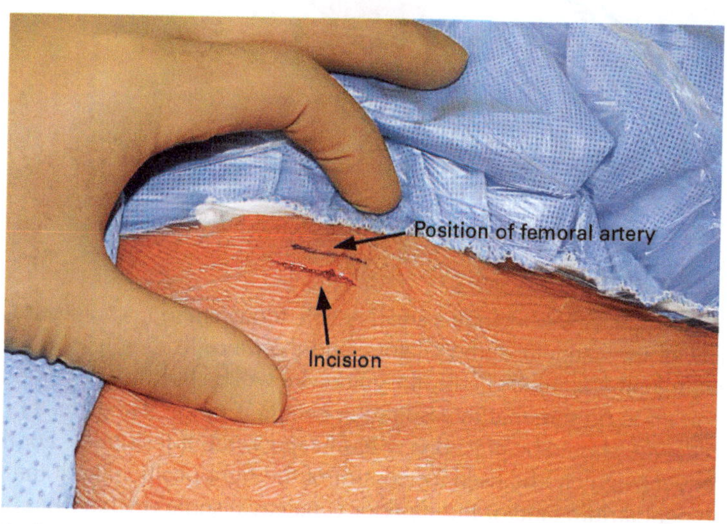

Fig. 4.1: The longitudinal incision is placed about 1 cm lateral to the femoral artery (marked here with a blue line).

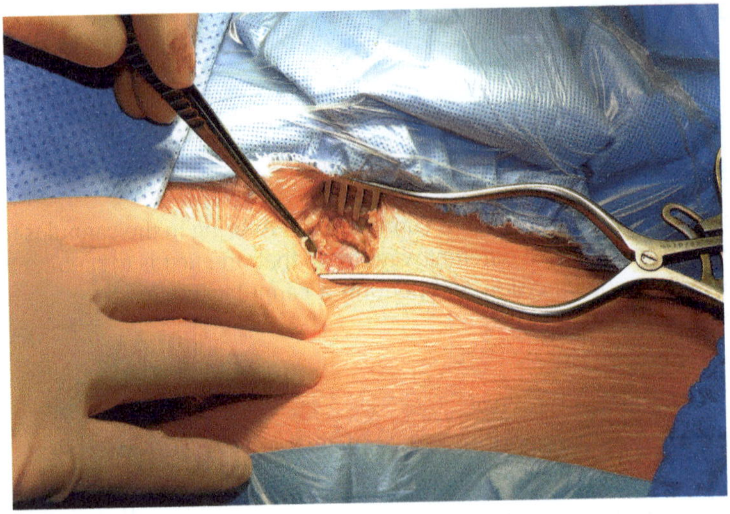

Fig. 4.2: Preparation of femoral vessels should allow the use of clamps in case of bleeding complications.

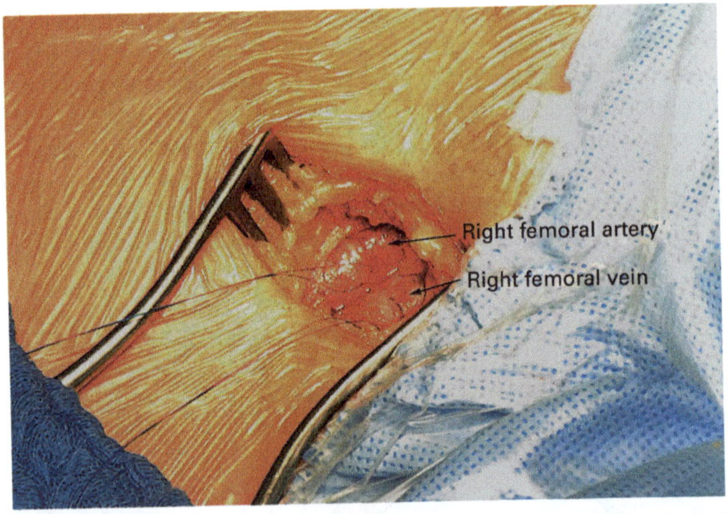

Fig. 4.3: Circular sutures for keeping the cannulas in position and closing the holes after removing the cannulas.

The usual introducer sets include a small needle for aspiration, a guidewire according to the length of the cannula, some dilators, and the inner leading part of the cannula. After aspiration with the small needle, the guidewire will be placed.

It is important to be sure that the aspiration needle is in the free diameter of the vessel. The guidewire should be placed very easily and without resistance. For the venous vessel a frequent sign can be used for control of the right positioning: If the guidewire reaches the right atrium (and/or the superior vena cava) some rhythm disturbances can be seen on the ECG monitor. The guidewire should be removed for a short distance – now it is placed perfectly.

The femoral vein is often found more posterior to the artery. So for technical reasons it is advantageous to start with the cannulation of the femoral vein.

Dilatation of the venous vessel is often not necessary. Normally the placement of the venous cannula over the right femoral vein is easy. The best way to reach this is the complete preparation of the adventitia at the point of cannula insertion. Sometimes it needs a very flexible cannula to pass through the abdominal part of the vessel, which means that, especially in cases of former abdominal operations, it can be difficult to reach the right atrium. In these cases (as in generally) the placement of the cannula should not be forced with a higher pressure at the end of the device. A change to the other side with preparation of the left femoral vein and the insertion of the cannula at this side should follow.

A fixation of the venous cannula after insertion is normally not necessary. The length of the cannula and the low venous blood pressure avoids the potential of the cannula slipping out of the vessel. Sometimes it is necessary to correct the cannula placement while the ECC is running to get a better blood evacuation. It is very easy to perform that when the cannula is not fixed.

The insertion of the arterial cannula is easier but can at times be more dangerous. To avoid problems, it is first important to be sure that the suture (and thus the insertion point for the cannula) is placed in a vessel region without calcifications. If there is some calcification the preparation should be enlarged to the proximal part of the vessel – never to the distal part. It is clear that a cannulation distal to a calcification or even a stenosis is not favorable for retrograde perfusion.

The general process of cannulation is not different from the practice in veins. After safely performed aspiration, a guidewire will be placed in the vessel. It is necessary to know that any resistance while forward moving of the guidewire is a clear signal to change the side and to use the left femoral artery. It depends on the type of cannula how far the tip of the cannula has to be placed inside the artery. The idea is not to bring in the arterial cannula as far as possible. In most types of cannulas it is absolutely enough to be sure that the first two or three centimeters are safe in the artery (▶Fig. 4.4). This avoids a higher danger of vessel perforation or wall injury and the worst case scenario with a retrograde arterial dissection after starting ECC.

If there is any suspicion for an arterial problem, an additional control step should be used. After starting ECC the pressure at the arterial line has to be monitored. If there is an abnormal increase while the first third of the perfusion flow is reached, two main reasons could be the primary cause. The first is a technical problem with the cannula itself. Sometimes there seems to be a variation in the inner diameter or the wall thickness of some arterial cannulas. Especially in higher flow rates, a smaller diameter leads to a relative higher flow resistance and to a higher flow pressure. This will be supported by a tight ligation of the cannula that is used for fixation. In general, a cannula with a preformed ligation ring seems to be advantageous.

The second reason could be an intimal flap that has been moved by the tip of the cannula in a central direction. After starting the ECC, a high flow resistance results in the danger of further damage to the intimal layer as a retrograde dissection. If there is any doubt about the correct function of the cannula the ECC must be stopped and the cannula has to be removed. Then the decision can be made to use the other side. It would be better and safer to switch from retrograde to antegrade perfusion. As a consequence, a direct cannulation of the ascending aorta must follow (see Chapter 5).

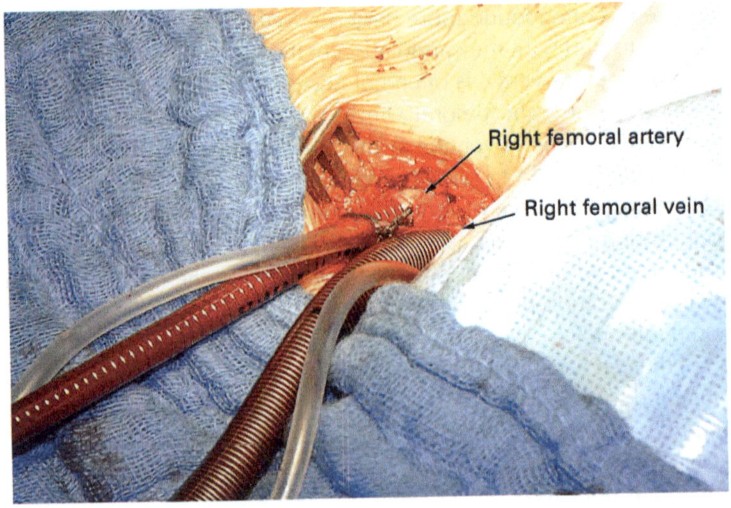

Fig. 4.4: Careful implantation of the arterial cannula. To avoid a perforation only the first few centimeters have to be brought in.

The fixation of the arterial cannula is a "must," of course. Similar to open heart surgery the arterial cannula falling out of the vessel is the absolute worst-case scenario after starting ECC. But in contrast to open heart surgery, with a safe reinsertion after stopping ECC with a very simple direct manipulation, the reimplantation of the cannula into the femoral artery can be a very confusing and time-consuming situation with a high danger for the patient. In general an arterial cannula with a specially formed ring at the outside of the device for fixation is recommended. These models avoid the narrowing of the cannula after fixation with a ligature.

4.1.2 Direct cannulation of the ascending aorta

In some cases the cannulation of the femoral artery is not possible. The reason might be known before the operation (as in cases of peripheral arterial disease) or can be shown after preparation of the vessels. Here, two consequences should be discussed: The first is the conversion of the operative method to an open heart procedure (which even should have been planned as such). The second is more elegant: a direct cannulation of the ascending aorta with a transthoracic access to the aorta or even directly through the right-lateral incision. Depending on the individual preferences of the surgeons, this kind of arterial cannulation might be the first choice for some. Because some rules regarding the ventilation of the patient have to be observed for retrograde perfusion, direct cannulation can have some advantages. In the end, the choice of arterial cannulation is also a question of what the surgeon has learned in the first place. Nevertheless, it must be a safe procedure and the surgeon has to feel comfortable with it.

To bring in the cannula through a transthoracic access it should be clear that the method of aortic cannulation is the same as in open heart surgery. This means one circular running suture and, for additional support after de-cannulation, an additional U-suture with pledgets at the ascending aorta (▶Fig. 4.5). Then, a stitch incision should

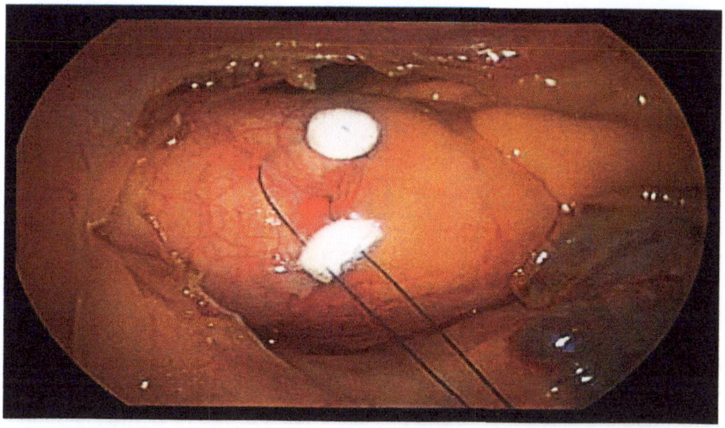

Fig. 4.5: Preparation for direct cannulation starts with a U-suture with pledgets.

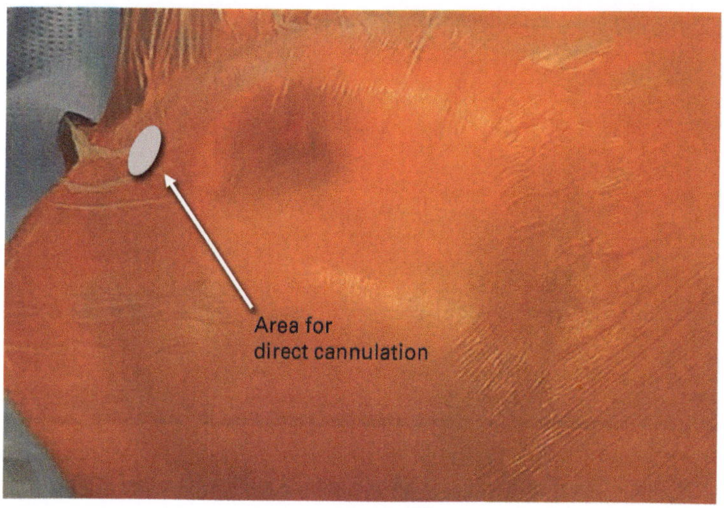

Fig. 4.6: A stitch incision in the second or third intercostal space (ICS) opens the way for the cannula directly into the thorax.

be performed in the second or third intercostal space (ICS) about 4 cm next to the sternum (▶Fig. 4.6). The ends of the running suture will be pulled out from the thoracic cavity through the incision and a snare will be brought in (▶Fig. 4.7).

Then, through the same incision, the cannula is pushed in immediately before the aortic wall. Under special check with the scope, a wall incision has to be made with the long knife. If the patient is older than age 50, this incision should be stopped before the inner layer is perforated (▶Fig. 4.8). In all other patients the incision should perforate all layers of the wall. The reason for this difference in procedure is the quality of the inner layer of the wall. In younger patients the layer is more elastic. This leads to very little bleeding only when the wall is perforated with a stitch. On the other side, if the inner layer is not perforated and the cannula is brought in, the risk of making a dissection is not low in these patients. In older patients there is normally a complete

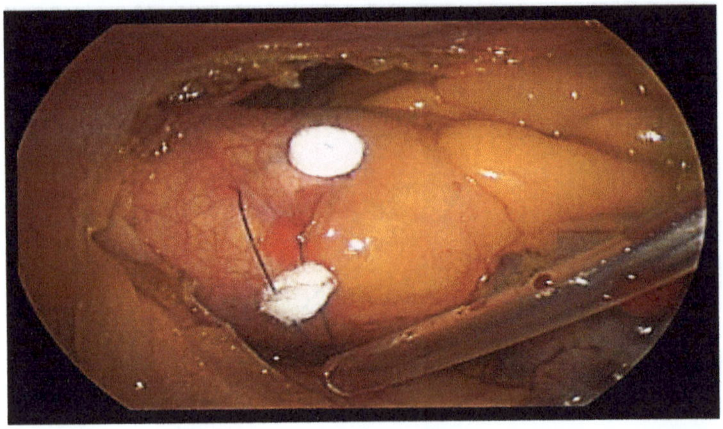

Fig. 4.7: The ends of the running suture come out of the thorax and a snare is brought in.

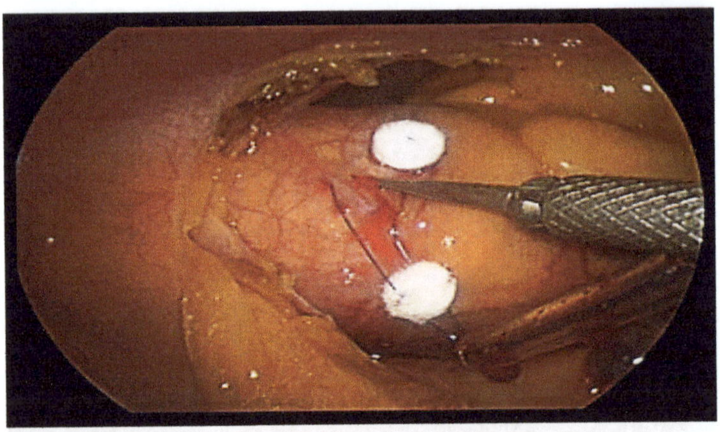

Fig. 4.8: The cannula has been brought in. The next step is the incision of the aortic wall with the long knife either through all layers (patients younger than age 50) or stopped before the inner layer (patients older than age 50).

opposite situation. Bleeding will be much higher after complete wall perforation and, because of the lower elastic layer, the risk of dissection is not as high.

Then the cannula has to be fixed about 2 cm above the tip of the cannula with a forceps in the right hand through the lateral thoracic incision. The next step is to push in the cannula with the left hand under, guiding the tip with the forceps. If the inner layer of the aortic wall has not been cut, the tip of the cannula should perforate the incised aortic wall and can be pushed forward into the ascending aorta (▶Fig. 4.9). The running suture will be snared and the cannula will be fixed with a ligature outside the thoracic cavity. The direct cannulation through the primary lateral mini-thoracotomy follows the same steps.

The main difference between the transthoracic and the direct cannulation is the way of the cannula from the thoracic cavity with either more (through the lateral incision) or no (through additional incision) restriction of the direct view and manipulation

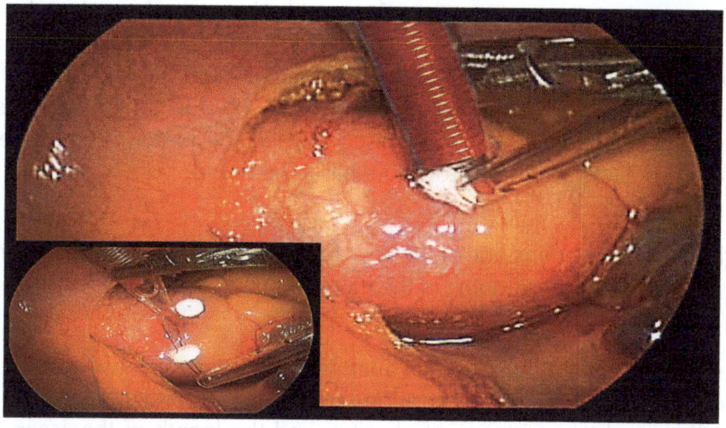

Fig. 4.9: The cannula was placed inside the aorta. In cases with a nonperforated inner layer, the tip of the cannula perforates it.

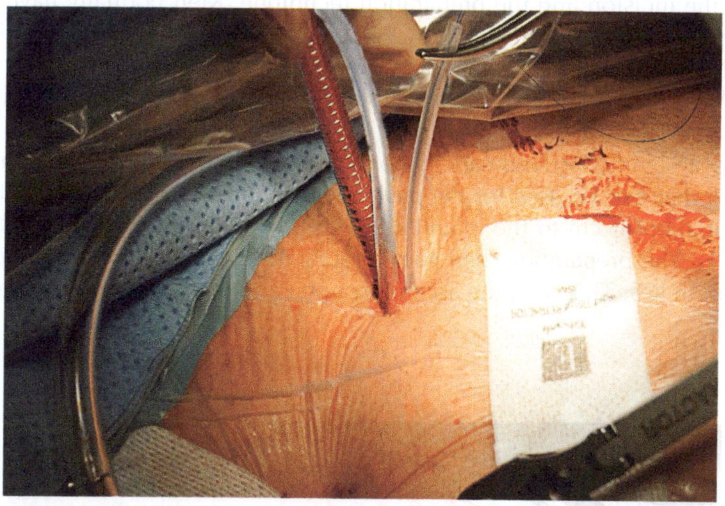

Fig. 4.10: If the cannula was brought in through an additional incision, the way to the valve is not restricted.

(▶Fig. 4.10). A larger lateral thoracotomy could help solve the problem of a direct cannulation, but actually the idea was not to have a longer incision.

4.2 Mini-thoracotomy

The discussion about the positioning and the length of the right-lateral incision might sometimes be a philosophical one. In reality, the choice of the access to the thoracic cavity is key for successful endoscopic surgery. It should be clear that the length of the incision is not a criterion for the quality of the operation, and there is no competition as to "who makes the shortest incision." In fact, the lateral positioning and the choice of the right intercostal space are the points of operation that most depend on the preferred individual set-up situation of the surgeon. However, the anatomy is nearly the same in every patient and some rules for this will be needed. On the other side, the length of the incision is one (but normally not the main) criterion for the patients in their decision-making process. So a compromise between the preferences of the surgeon and the idea of a real endoscopic procedure has to be found.

The right-lateral incision is one of the keys for successful endoscopic surgery. It is not the length but the positioning of the incision that makes the difference.

In respect to the variability of normal anatomy, the distance between the lower thoracic orifice and the shoulder, the position of the right diaphragm (which follows the size of the liver and the existence of obesity), and the length of the ascending aorta have an important influence on the localization of the skin incision.

The anatomical differences between men and women are other criteria for the choice of the incision and the preparation technique. Men normally have a longer longitudinal axis of the thorax and women a shorter one. However, in obese patients the right diaphragm can reach the middle of the thorax in both men and women. As a consequence, the space inside the thorax can be very small in these cases.

There is a significant landmark for orientation in men. The right mamilla is a benchmark that can be used for the positioning of the incision. Normally I prefer a distance of about 3 cm to the mamilla where I make an incision of about 3–4 cm (▶Fig. 4.11). The preparation then goes directly through the fatty and muscle tissue and the fourth ICS. This way, the ascending aorta and the left atrium can be reached very easily.

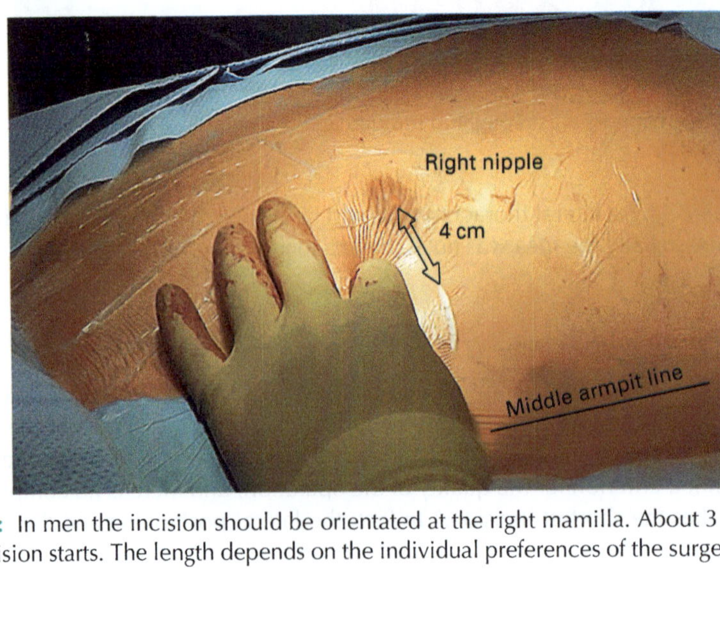

Fig. 4.11: In men the incision should be orientated at the right mamilla. About 3 cm next to it the incision starts. The length depends on the individual preferences of the surgeon.

In men the mamilla is the landmark for orientation. A short incision about 3 cm next to the mamilla leads to a preparation through the fourth ICS to open the right pleural space.

In women the same incision as in men would cut through the breast, which is not a good idea and, therefore, we have to adapt the localization of the skin incision to realize the thoracic access through the fourth ICS. The consequence is an incision about 1 cm above the breast fold (this is roughly above the fifth or sometimes the sixth ICS) in the same length as in men (▶Fig. 4.12). This localization has two advantages: First, there is a cosmetic aspect because at the end nothing of the scare will be seen. Second, the woman with such a scar will not have any problems with the use of underwear. All these ideas may seem unimportant. However, remember that we want to operate on these patients at an early stage of the disease with fewer symptoms. The attention of these matters of minor importance may help to come to a better individual decision.

In women the incision should be made 1 cm above the breast fold. After preparation upward, the opening of the right thoracic cavity is performed in the fourth ICS just as in men.

Then the incision has to go through the fatty tissue until the muscle layer is reached. Then the preparation has to go upward along the muscle layer until it reaches the fourth ICS. Opening the thoracic cavity follows the standard procedure, as in men.

In some cases with obesity and/or liver enlargement, the right part of the diaphragm will be found directly after opening the thoracic cavity in the fourth ICS (▶Fig. 4.13). In these cases both a direct view to the valve and the use of the instruments might be reduced. Here, a 2–0 suture can help, which goes through the tip of the diaphragm (Be careful of the liver: avoid a deeper stitch than 2–3 mm) after insertion of the rib retractor. Then, the tip of the diaphragm can be pulled back to the intercostal incision and

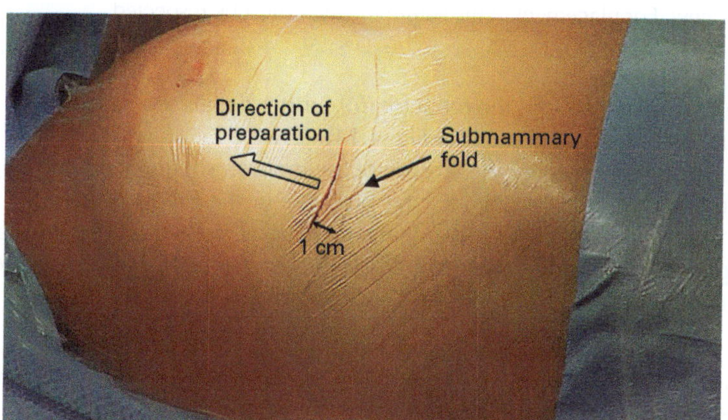

Fig. 4.12: In women the incision should be placed about 1 cm above the breast fold. To go through the fourth ICS, a preparation from this point up to the fourth ICS must be carried out.

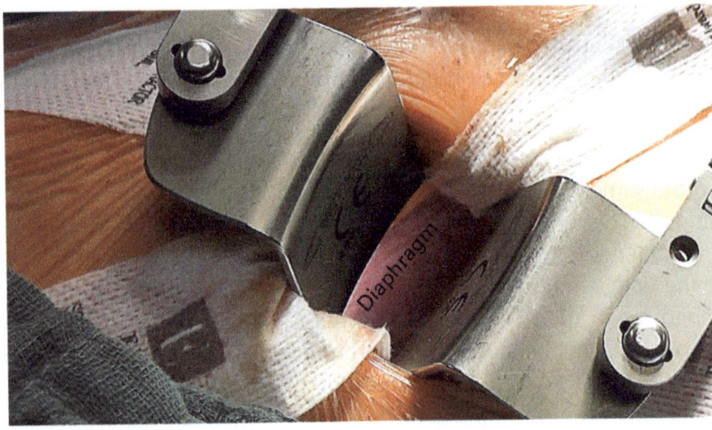

Fig. 4.13: Typical situation in patients with a very high right diaphragm because of obesity. The way to the valve is significantly obstructed.

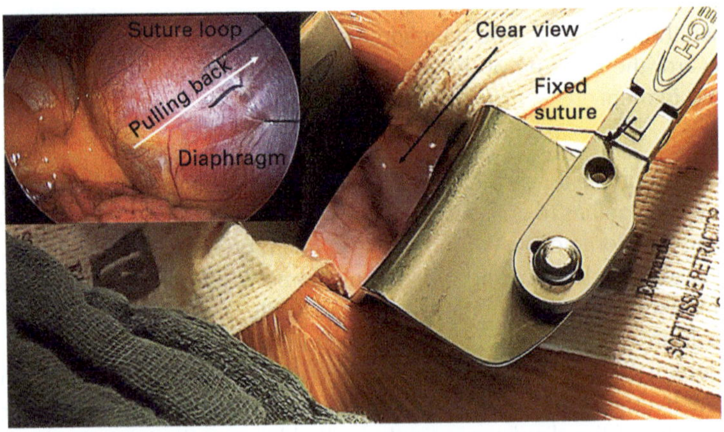

Fig. 4.14: With a suture through the highest point, the diaphragm can be pulled back and kept out of view. For placement of the suture the liver must be respected.

the suture can be tied around the retractor (for further details see Section 6.2). Then the view should be as clear as possible (▶Fig. 4.14).

At the end of the procedure the closure of the incision should include a single adaptation suture for the ribs to avoid a lung prolapse in the follow-up period. A double injection of a long-lasting and local analgetic drug at both wound poles has proved itself for preventing postoperative wound pain (see also Section 2.2). The rest of the wound will be closed layer for layer in a normal standard technique.

A suture through the tip of the diaphragm can be used for retrieving the diaphragm out of the direct view and the way of instruments.

4.3 Ports

The use of ports in combination with a mini-thoracotomy is a compromise between complete endoscopic surgery and the necessity of direct access to the mitral valve. Nevertheless, the use of ports can help the work in a clearly defined setup with excellent opportunities for the instruments' way in and out. These ports for instruments should have a diameter of 10 mm for comfortable working and the opportunity to bring in a suture through the port if necessary.

Another necessity for the use of ports is the videoscopic camera. Here, a size-adapted port should be used for a largely atraumatic transthoracic way of the videoscopic system. Because of the sometimes small ICS it seems to be advantageous to use a 5 mm optical system with a 5 mm port. Here, the danger for injuries of intercostal arteries is low.

At minimum for that idea, an exact positioning of the port is absolutely necessary. First, the right position of the port depends on the decision for a 0° optical system or even a 30° system. The main difference results from the opportunity of a 30° system to "look around." This means the possibility to rotate both the endoscopic picture on the screen with a rotation of the optical camera and the direction of the view with a rotation of the 30° optical lens (for details see Section 4.4). That way, getting an endoscopic view on the valve (or even on the right thoracic cavity) leads over the introduction of the optical system beside the direction of the direct view until a point where the valve can be seen with a 30° rotated lens.

As a consequence, the port of the camera can be placed a bit more to the anterior and upper part of the right thoracic wall than the mini-thoracotomy. To place the port optimally in the second or third ICS about 6–7 cm from the sternum and about at the same level as the mini-thoracotomy, a stitch incision has to be made (▶Fig. 4.15).

For the use of instrumental ports, a virtual triangle should imagine with the tip about 4 cm behind the mini-thoracotomy, the left pole that results from the videoscopic port and the right pole at the same level as the mini-thoracotomy but in the sixth ICS (▶Fig. 4.16). Such a setup would be another technical prerequisite for complete endoscopic surgery.

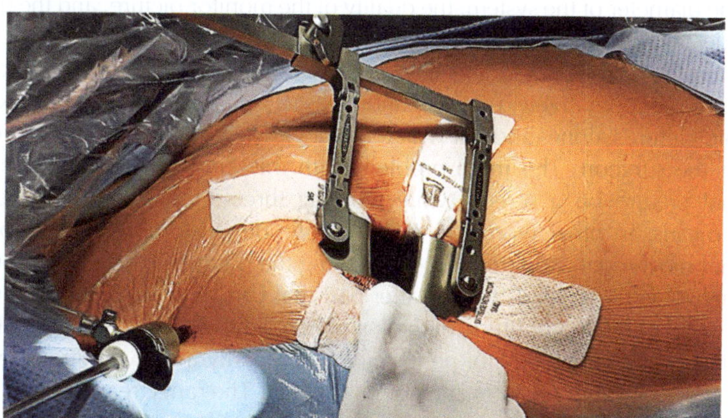

Fig. 4.15: Typical placement of a 5 mm port for the videoscope with a 30° optical system. For a 0° system the position should be changed more to the thoracic incision.

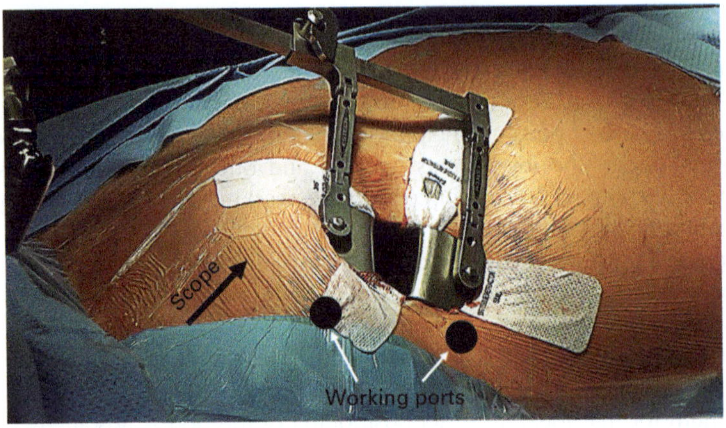

Fig. 4.16: For working with ports alone, a different placement of ports has to be chosen. This is the prerequisite for complete endoscopic surgery.

Ports are helpful to get atraumatic access to the thorax for videoscope and instruments; they are necessary for complete endoscopic surgery. The position of every single port must be adapted to the optical system and the type of work.

4.4 Videoscopy

Before starting the discussion about the technique of videoscopy and the use of optical systems in endoscopic mitral valve surgery, it should be clarified that the issue of this chapter is not the technical background or the description of the technical details of different optical systems. That issue is left to industrial suppliers.

Discussing videoscopy means describing all the details of use that can be important for successful endoscopic surgery. This includes the question of the optical wrinkle of viewing, the diameter of the system, the quality of the monitor picture, and the discussion of helpful details.

A general preliminary remark has to be made about the role of videoscopic pictures as a part of intraoperatively used technologies. The contribution of working with videoscopic pictures alone (and not with a direct view) depends on the experience and training of the surgeon. The main problem with this kind of work is seeing a two-dimensional picture on a screen while working three-dimensionally inside the left atrium. It means, in other words, to realize a two-dimensional picture into a three-dimensional movement. Additionally, magnifying the picture on screen in comparison with the native situation leads to a smaller part that can be seen than in a direct view with a seemingly higher amplitude of the instrumental movements. Because of that, the role of videoscopic technology for performing a minimally invasive mitral valve reconstruction differs substantially from surgeon to surgeon. The range reaches from surgeons that perform nearly all manipulations at the valve with videoscopic pictures alone (like me) to surgeons that use the videoscopic system for lighting only. It should be clear that in the last case a greater lateral thoracic incision is the prerequisite.

The greatest advantage, and the point that speaks most for working with endoscopic pictures, is the excellent depiction of details at both the valve level and the level underneath the valve. Especially for implantation of artificial chords, the surgeon will find bright lighting and detailed pictures of the left ventricular cavity, which make it much easier. For working on the valve itself the videoscopic picture is very helpful (and sometimes the only possibility to work) in patients with an unfavorable anatomical situation.

Using a videoscope helps get an excellent overview of the details of the valve. It allows the surgeon to see all parts of the valve that cannot be seen directly.

4.4.1 The wrinkle

After these remarks, the wrinkle at the tip of the camera should be discussed. In general there are two different systems on the market: a system with a direction of 0° and a system with 30°. The quality of the monitor pictures is the same. But it is easy to imagine that a 0° system needs a nearly direct orientation of the whole camera to the valve whereas a 30° system has to come in from a direction at the side of the direct view (with a difference of about 30° to the direct view, of course). As a consequence, a 30° system is more comfortable because only the tip is seen in the direct view (▶Fig. 4.17).

For practical use these considerations are important to develop an uncomplicated and repeatable setup. In the end, the main goal of an acceptable setup should be a situation with a clear way for the instruments, an acceptable direct view (if necessary), and an excellent endoscopic view without any obstruction. For the use of an optical system it means that a 30° system is more advantageous than a 0° system.

Using a 30° optical system has the advantage of keeping the scope out of the direct view. Additionally, it allows checking a large part of the inner side of the thoracic wall.

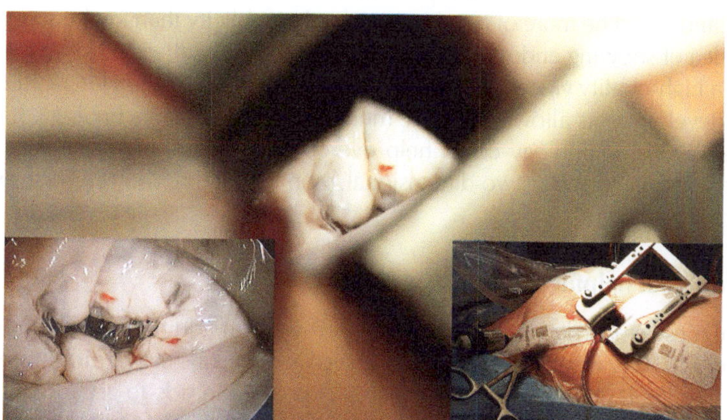

Fig. 4.17: Using a 30° optical system means seeing only the tip of the scope in a direct view. The way to the valve is not blocked.

Another aspect of a 30° system is the possibility to check a large area of the thoracic wall from the inner side, which means having control over bleeding and avoiding a re-thoracotomy in many cases. The different opportunities for changing the view with the three-dimensional movement of the camera itself and the side-orientated lens of the camera allows a complete view to the thoracic wall. Additionally, with the rotation of the head of the camera, a circular view is reached.

4.4.2 The diameter

For general use of the optical system it does not matter what diameter the camera has because the optical characteristics are the same. It can be said that a 10 mm system is more stable and not so sensitive to movements.

But a 10 mm system means a 10 mm port with a larger hole. In smaller patients the ICS is sometimes smaller than 10 mm, and in these cases a 10 mm system leads to pressure on the ribs during surgery and can result in a long-lasting irritation of the periosteum.

So, in the end, if there is the opportunity to choose between the systems the thinner one should be chosen. After the first experience with a 5 mm system it will never be changed.

> A 5 mm optical system has no limitations in comparison to a 10 mm one. The advantage is that a smaller port is needed, which helps avoid both bleeding complications and postoperative pain.

4.4.3 The monitor picture

Technical developments lead us to the best possible picture. In the end, it means that today, high definition (HD) technology is the standard for high quality. But it should be clear that a technical background and instruments are expensive, and for successful endoscopic surgery an HD picture is not the absolute condition. If there is a good-quality magnified videoscopic picture of the valve, the additional advantage of an HD picture will be very small and could be more of a technology for the publicity than for the surgeon. However, the idea of showing endoscopic pictures to a group of colleagues or in a meeting or to receive a high-quality video documentation may lead to a decision for an HD system.

Recent developments allow seeing the monitor picture in 3D technology. It is still unclear whether this technology could help overcome the discrepancy between a three-dimensional working and a two-dimensional monitor picture, but the first experience looks promising.

4.4.4 Additional helpful details

The first of these small details is the use of a port with an additional opportunity for the insufflation of CO_2. For both the resterilizable and the one-way-articles are different models on the market with an additional small cock at the side to get a junction with a CO_2 line (▶Fig. 4.18).

The second detail is the use of a small cleaning paper for the tip of the camera. It is often necessary to clean the camera while it is moving or while the instruments cause a

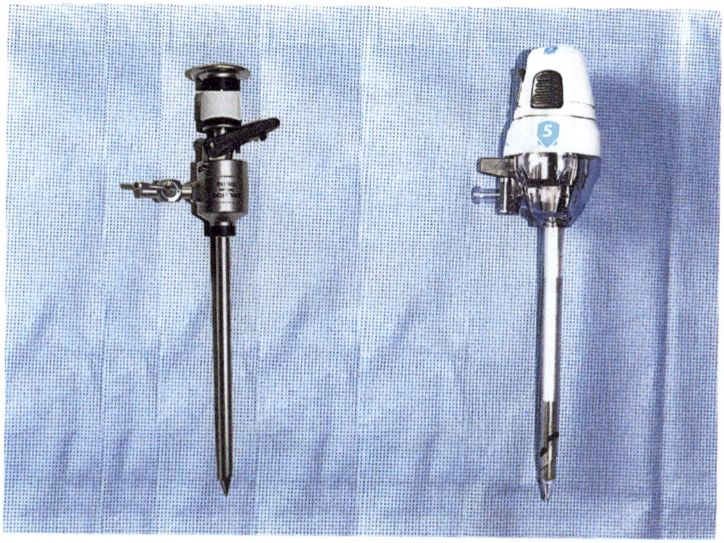

Fig. 4.18: Examples for ports that are being used for videoscopes with an additional connector for a CO_2 line. Both single-use and resterilizable models are available on the market.

pollution of the tip. Here, a prepared cleaning paper is on the market that combines a fluid for cleaning and a feature to avoid growing moldy (▶Fig. 4.19).

Warming the tip of the scope before the first use helps avoid a foggy monitor picture as well as the use of cleaning papers.

Normally the temperature inside the operating room is lower than 37°C. If the scope has this temperature when it is introduced into the thoracic cavity the monitor picture will quickly appear foggy. To avoid this, the scope has to warm up before introducing it. An electrical device can be bought for camera warming or even a simple bowl with warm water might be enough to warm up the tip of the scope.

4.5 Cardioplegia

It is beyond the scope of this work to discuss the different technologies and cardioplegic solutions to induce cardiac arrest. Nevertheless, the use of cardioplegia should be a "must" in mitral valve surgery. The only exception is the redo-operation in patients with former aortocoronary bypass grafting or aortic valve procedures. This will be discussed later in this chapter (see Section 4.5.2).

4.5.1 Use of cardioplegia

The first decision that has to be made is whether to choose antegrade or retrograde perfusion of the coronary arteries. Because of technical reasons it is recommended that an

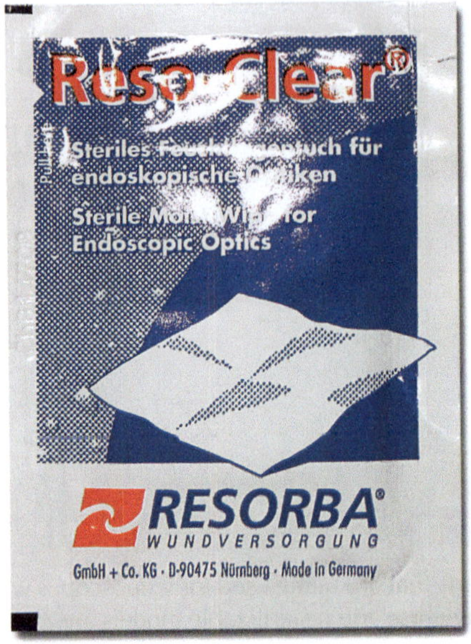

Fig. 4.19: Cleaning paper for a videoscope, which helps avoid a foggy monitor and cleans the tip of the scope from blood and tissue.

antegrade perfusion with an injection into the aortic root is used. Here, two different techniques are in use.

The first option is a single-shot technique with a steel needle directly into the root, removing the needle when cardioplegic solution is given (▶Fig. 4.20). The advantage is a good control of the aspiration and simple handling. The hole in the aortic wall can be closed immediately after removing the needle or after declamping the aorta. However, there are two great disadvantages. The use of a single-shot technique means that in cases of a longer time of reconstruction with a longer time of cardiac arrest, an additional cardioplegic shot could be necessary. In this case, another aspiration of the aortic root must follow and in most cases the same hole will not pierced. In the end there is an additional potential reason for bleeding. The other fact is the disability of active de-airing of the aortic root before declamping the aorta. The result might be a higher risk of cerebral air embolism.

> The single-shot technique with an immediately removable needle is easy to perform and safe. But the disadvantages, such as a problematic second shot or the impossibility of an active de-airing, make it a second choice.

The second option is the use of a system that is fixed after aspiration of the root, which stays there during the whole ECC. To reach this situation, at first a U-suture with pledgets should be placed where the needle will be pushed in. This suture is used for closing the hole at the end only and should be positioned at the upper quarter of aortic

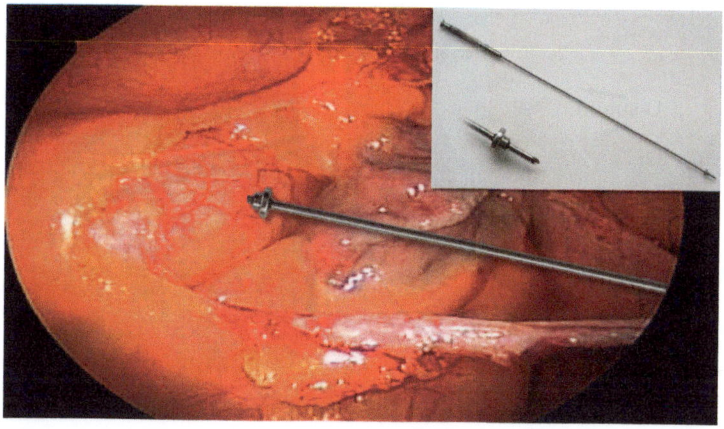

Fig. 4.20: Single-shot technique for application of cardioplegia via a steel needle. After removal of the needle an active de-airing of the aortic root is no longer possible.

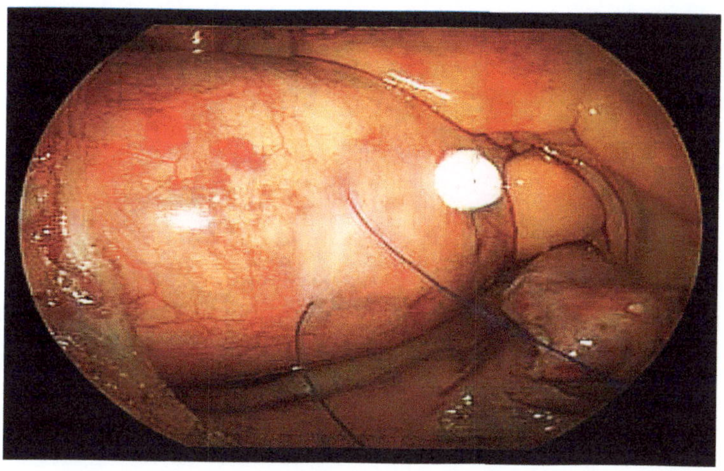

Fig. 4.21: A U-suture for closing the aspiration hole at the end (after de-airing of the root) has to be placed at the lateral wall of the aorta.

circumference (▶Fig. 4.21). In the middle of that area, an additional suture for fixation of the cardioplegic system is placed. The ends of this suture will be led through the small holes of the holding system at the tip of the needle in a crossover technique (▶Fig. 4.22), and the needle will be led in as on splints. After aspiration, in the middle of the U-suture area, the needle will be fixed with knots (▶Fig. 4.23).

After that procedure, the guiding stick can be removed under clamping the system. The free end of the cardioplegic cannula should be led out through the same stitch incision that will be used later for the aortic clamp. Then, a three-way cock should be used for the connection to the cardioplegic line and for a second line for suction. So, at first, the cardioplegic solution can be administered and should be repeated for multiple shots of cardioplegia. In the end, with an easy switch of the three-way cock the suction will support de-airing the aortic root (▶Fig. 4.24).

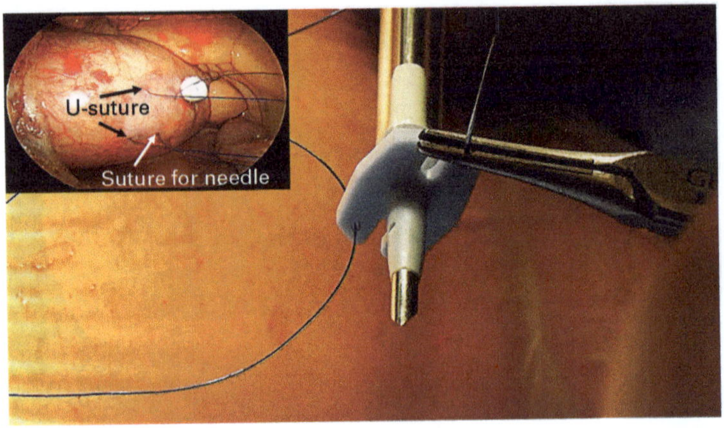

Fig. 4.22: An additional suture for keeping the system in position has to be placed (see insert) and leads through the small holes of the system.

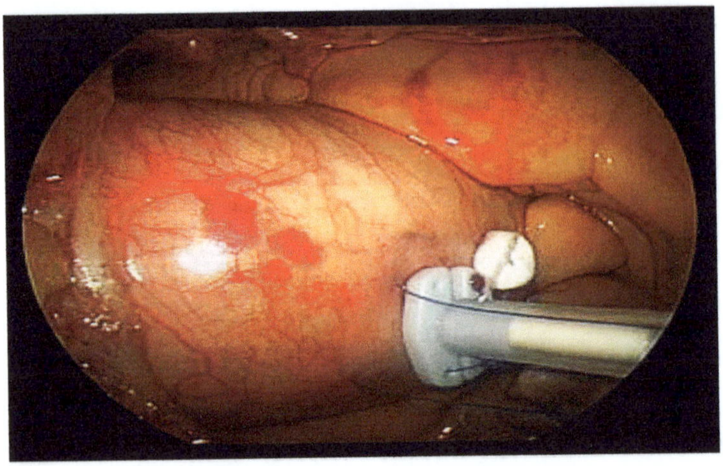

Fig. 4.23: The system is positioned in the aorta and the suture is tied.

> The use of a fixable cardioplegic system with the opportunity to reach both a multiple cardioplegic shot and an active de-airing of the aortic root should be the procedure of choice.

The cardioplegic system can be removed under the conditions of an unloaded heart immediately before the ECC is weaned. The U-suture will be used for closing the hole in the aortic wall. It is important to check the aspiration area under normal blood pressure. In every case of minimal bleeding, a second suture should be placed to be sure that there is no risk for the patient.

For the procedure of removing the system, there is a little trick to avoid too much bleeding out of the hole. After cutting the fixation suture using the U-suture, one knot

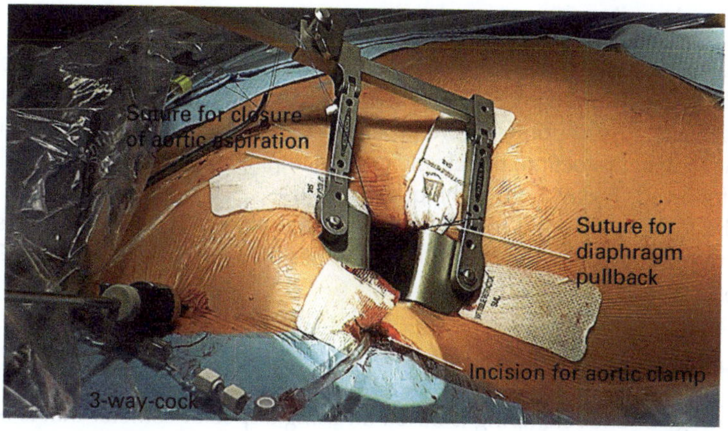

Fig. 4.24: After removing the guiding needle, the free end of the system is led out of the thorax through the incision that was made for aortic clamping. Over a three-way stop cock, cardioplegic shots and de-airing of the root are possible.

should be prepared and should be pushed in with the knot pusher before the needle is removed. Then the needle can be removed from the aorta with the left hand, which holds one end of the suture, and so in the moment when the needle is outside the aorta the knot can be tied using the knot pusher in the right hand.

4.5.2 Operations under fibrillation

Another option is to carry out the operation without any cardioplegia. In these cases the permanent fibrillation of the heart leads to the opportunity to open the left atrium when the heart is unloaded and no blood will be ejected. For practical use, it is important to know that there are some disadvantages. Without concentration on the details much more intra-atrial bleeding, a lower quality of viewing, a higher risk of air embolism, and a more complicated reconstruction technique can be listed.

Because of these reasons the technology without the use of cardioplegia should be reserved for redo-cases only. Here, a structural problem of the valve is rare. The reason for mitral valve regurgitation is very often a dilated native ring in combination with more or less restriction of the posterior leaflet. As a consequence the implantation of an artificial ring is in many of these cases the procedure of choice (sometimes in combination with the cut of some secondary chords). So we often find a relatively easier reconstruction procedure and can carry it out under the unfavorable condition of a fibrillated heart in most of these cases.

> Operations without cardioplegia should be reserved for redo procedures only. In these cases most repairs of the mitral valve can be performed with the implantation of an artificial ring only.

4.6 Aortic clamping

From the very beginning of the development of an endoscopic mitral valve technology, the so-called endoclamping was the main idea to get an aortic occlusion and to induce cardioplegia. Because of some severe problems (balloon movement, aortic dissection, insufficient cardiac protection) the classic cross clamping as an alternative idea for aortic clamping followed. Today, both techniques are in use.

Here, the focus is directed to the detailed description of the modified classic cross clamping that was named after its main developer, Randy Chitwood, as the Chitwood technique.

4.6.1 Endoclamping

The technology of endoclamping is based on using a special catheter that is brought in over the femoral artery. This catheter has different lumina and a balloon near the tip (▶Fig. 4.25). It allows inflating the balloon after it is placed in the ascending aorta and inducing cardioplegia proximal to this balloon simultaneously. The inflation of the balloon "seals" the ascending aorta from the inner side.

The procedure of endoclamping seems to be relatively simple. In experienced hands and in routine use it might be reliable and safe. But some disadvantages such as the possibility of balloon movement, the necessity for a continuous check of the correct position by TEE, the risk of developing an aortic dissection, and the uncontrolled retrograde way over the aortic arch make this procedure not the first choice for aortic clamping at the beginning of endoscopic mitral surgery.

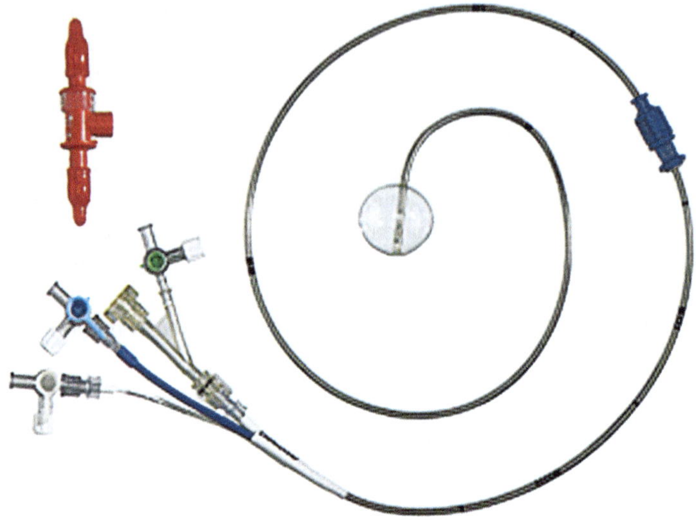

Fig. 4.25: Typical example of a catheter for endoclamping. Different lumina allow inflating and deflating the balloon at the tip and inducing cardioplegia simultaneously (Edwards Lifesciences; Irvine, CA, USA).

4.6.2 The Chitwood technique

The main principle of the Chitwood technique is similar to the cross clamping we know from open heart surgery. A clamp is used that completely and safely seals the aorta. However, in contrast to open heart surgery the branches of the clamp reach the aorta not from the back but from the side. This seemingly banal difference marks some important aspects of that technique.

For the use of the clamp an additional small incision is necessary. It should be made in the anterior armpit line where the third ICS is located (▶Fig. 4.26). As described, this incision can be used for leading out of the cardioplegia line (see also Section 4.5).

For the Chitwood technique, clamps with three different lengths of the branches are available. Normally it is enough to choose between the clamp with the shortest and the medium-length branches (▶Fig. 4.27). The necessity of these different clamps results from the different diameters of the aorta (shorter branches could be too short for a larger aortic diameter) but will be limited through the space inside the thorax. It is easy to imagine that the longer the branches of the clamp the space will grow up that is needed inside for opening.

> Aortic clamps after Chitwood allow cross clamping the aorta as in open heart surgery. The main difference is the direction of the clamp that comes from the side instead of the back.

The second main technical aspect is the curve of the branches. This is necessary to avoid injuries to structures on the left side of the aorta. The clamp should be closed with branches bent upward (i.e., to the aortic arch).

It has become apparent that the clamp has to be introduced with branches bent downward (i.e., with the tip to the diaphragm). A 180° rotation before the aorta is reached seems to be the best way to avoid complications (now the tip is directed upward to the aortic arch).

Under check with a direct view or with the videoscopic camera, the aorta now can be raised a bit with the forceps and the posterior branch (remember: it is bent upward)

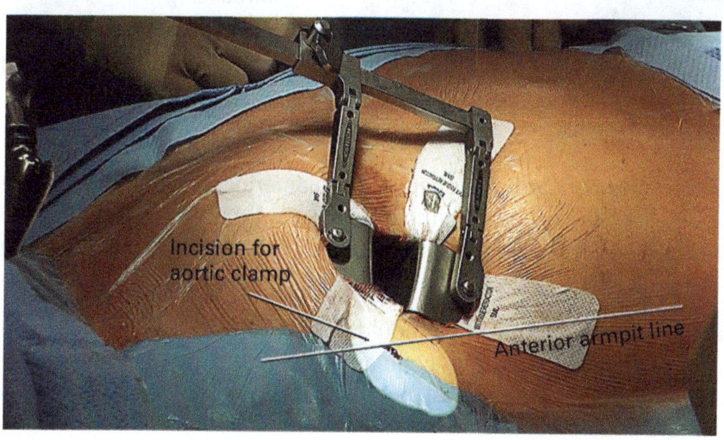

Fig. 4.26: Position of the incision for the aortic clamp in the anterior armpit line.

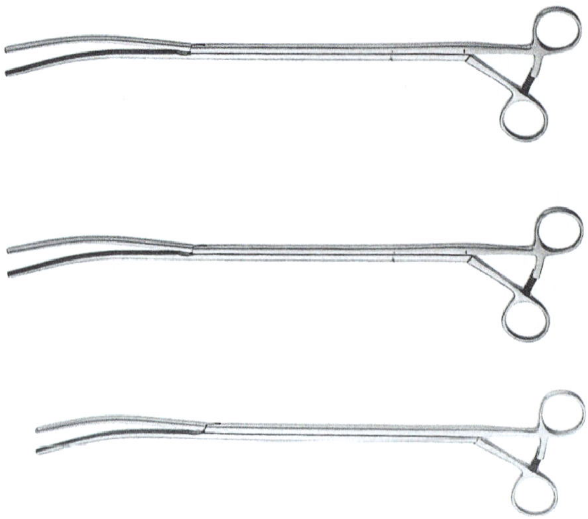

Fig. 4.27: Typical examples of aortic clamps according to Chitwood's model. Normally the smallest and the medium-sized one are enough for all situations (Estech, San Ramon, CA, USA).

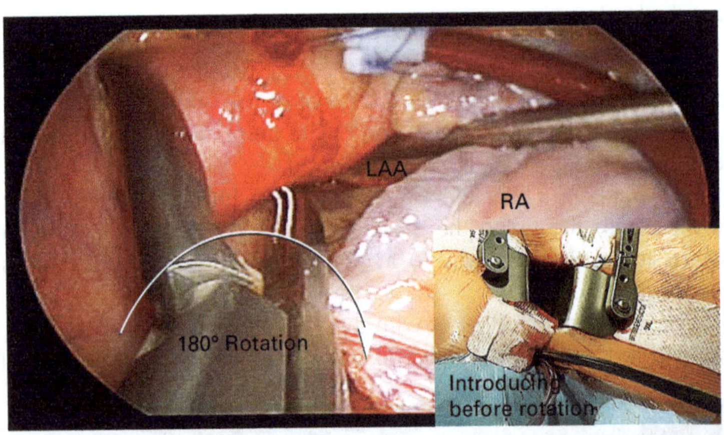

Fig. 4.28: The aortic clamp is placed and the branches can be closed. It is clear that the tip of the branches show to the aortic arch after a rotation of 180°.

can be placed. If the pericardium is between the anterior branch and the aorta it can be pushed away with the forceps. Then the clamp can be pushed carefully forward as is necessary. When the situation is checked again the clamp can be closed (▶Fig. 4.28).

The curve of the clamp branches should have a direction to the heart when the clamp will be brought in. But to avoid an injury of left-sided tissue (the left atrial appendage) a 180° rotation must be carried out before the branches will be placed before and behind the aorta.

4.6.3 Complications

The cross clamping under the use of Chitwood's technology is relatively simple to carry out. However, because of the central meaning for the endoscopic procedure it needs special attention. This central meaning particularly results from the disastrous consequences for another operation if an injury of the pulmonary artery or of the left atrial appendage is caused by the use of the clamp. In both cases a bleeding results that is normally not supplied through an endoscopic access. A larger anterolateral incision or the conversion to a sternotomy must follow.

The main reason for bleeding out of the left atrial appendage is the false rotation of the clamp and thus a perforation of the wall of the left atrial appendage. Since the perforation cannot be felt (there is not really a resistance) the only way to avoid this problem is to avoid false rotation.

However, perforation of a pulmonary artery develops differently. Here, a resistance often can be felt before the vessel is perforated in the end. To avoid this situation the position of the clamp and the diameter of the aorta should be checked very carefully and the clamp should not be pushed against any resistance. If there is any resistance the clamp should be pulled back and a new attempt to place the clamp has to be made under verified conditions.

A bleeding out of the pulmonary artery or the left atrial appendage must be avoided. Normally these complications cannot be supplied through a mini-thoracotomy.

Sometimes bleeding out of the left atrial appendage might only be seen after declamping the aorta and after filling the heart, that is, at the end of a sometimes time-consuming and complicated reconstruction. As a consequence, this will lead to a conversion to stop the bleeding after the surgeon has successfully finished the main part of the operation. It demonstrates the importance of careful clamping for the overall success of an endoscopic procedure. Otherwise, this is one of the most unsatisfactory situations for the surgeon.

Remember: To avoid these two complications it is only necessary to rotate the clamp after introducing and to check very attentively the depth to which the clamp was pushed.

5 Valve repair techniques

The following explains the basic knowledge to describe a mitral valve. Hence, the reader that is familiar with this special code may jump to the next chapter.

Talking about mitral valve repair techniques means having a common language to describe findings and technologies. This is necessary not only to discuss from surgeon to surgeon but also from surgeons to cardiologists. The exact description of a finding of a functional mitral valve problem by a cardiologist can be translated into the exact planning of a repair by the surgeon.

To achieve this, the well-known anatomical structures of the valve are not enough. A more functional view describes the different parts of the leaflets in a nomenclature that orientates from the left to the right when the view comes from the atrial side. The anterior leaflet is divided into three parts called A1 to A3. Correspondingly, the posterior leaflet is divided into three parts too, but is, of course, named P1 to P3 (▶Fig. 5.1).

5.1 Quadrangular resection

One of the most needed repair techniques is the quadrangular resection of a part of the prolapsed leaflet. This technique is similar to triangular resection, a repair technique that helps in many cases of a localized prolapse at the segments P1 to P3.

5.1.1 Pathological anatomy

The typical finding for using this technique is an enlarged and prolapsed part of the posterior leaflet. For planning the repair it is necessary to understand that there is

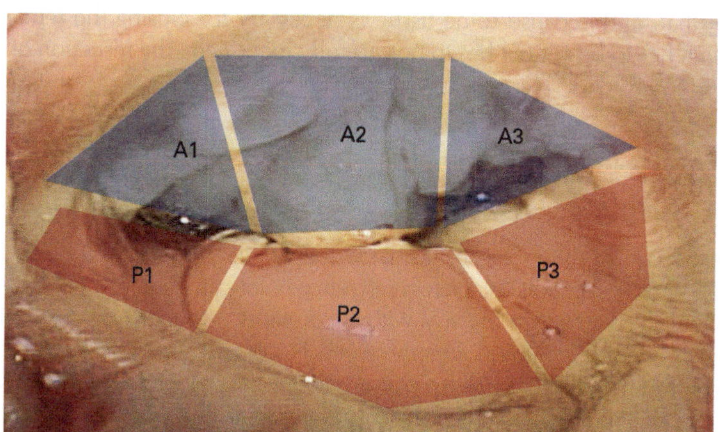

Fig. 5.1: Anterior and posterior leaflets are divided into three parts. The anterior parts are named A1 to A3 and the posterior parts are correspondingly named P1 to P3.

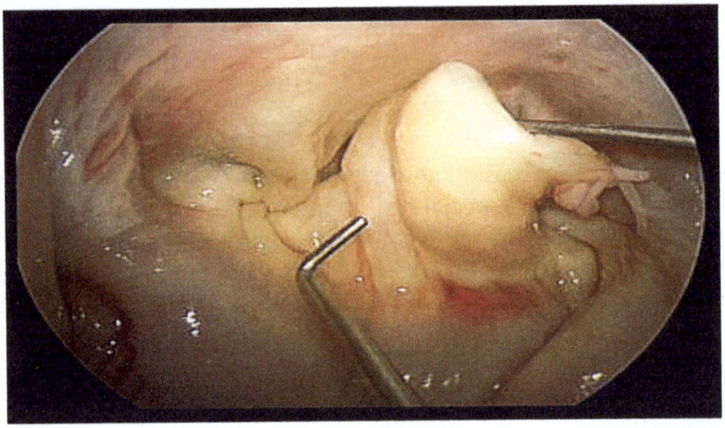

Fig. 5.2: Limited prolapse of the middle posterior segment. This is the typical finding that allows a simple quadrangular or triangular resection.

an area of the posterior leaflet with too much tissue and elongated and/or ruptured chords (▶Fig. 5.2). As a consequence, there is a leaflet that is too high at this point and that will show a systolic movement into the left atrium. Although for using the technique described here the area of prolaptic tissue normally includes one segment, only sometimes this area is very large indeed and includes half or more than half of the posterior leaflet (▶Fig. 5.3). In these cases another technology (neochord insertion, sliding plastic) or a combination of more than one technique is necessary.

5.1.2 Theoretical remarks

The idea to repair this situation is to cut out a part of the prolapsed tissue. In respect to the finding of mostly one included segment, a narrowing of the annulus follows routinely. The lateral parts of the prolapse often have chords with an acceptable function. Because of that, and because some tissue is necessary for closing the remaining gap, the tissue that has to be cut out has to be carefully identified. The resection of too much tissue has to be avoided.

5.1.3 Practical realization

Identifying the prolapse

First, the extension of the prolapse has to be identified. With the two nerve hooks the examination starts at segment A1. Here a reference point can often be defined. At least all segments were checked and so the area with the prolapse is found very easily (▶Fig. 5.4).

After identifying the prolapsed area the extension of the resection should be defined. For that the middle part is lifted with a nerve hook so that the prolapse area is spread out (▶Fig. 5.5). With the other hook the free edge is pulled back step by step to both sides. If the edge can be pulled back there is still prolaptic tissue. If a resistance can be noticed at the level of the valve then functional acceptable conditions are reached. The transition between these two findings defines the limits of the prolapse very well (▶Fig. 5.6).

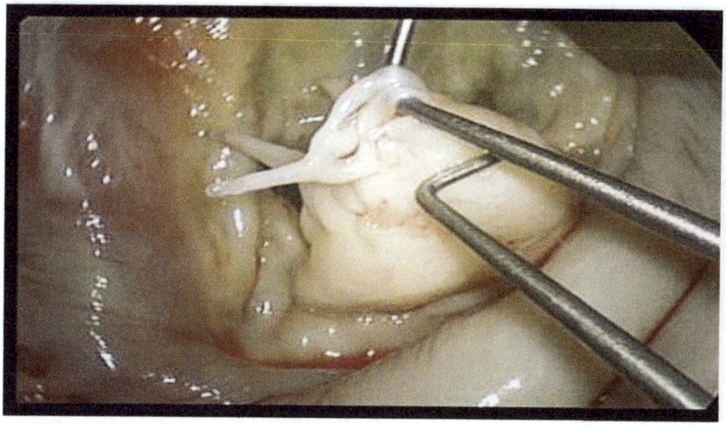

Fig. 5.3: Large prolapse of the posterior leaflet that includes all posterior segments. In these cases a simple quadrangular or triangular resection is not possible or not enough. For a stable repair a combination of more than one method is often necessary.

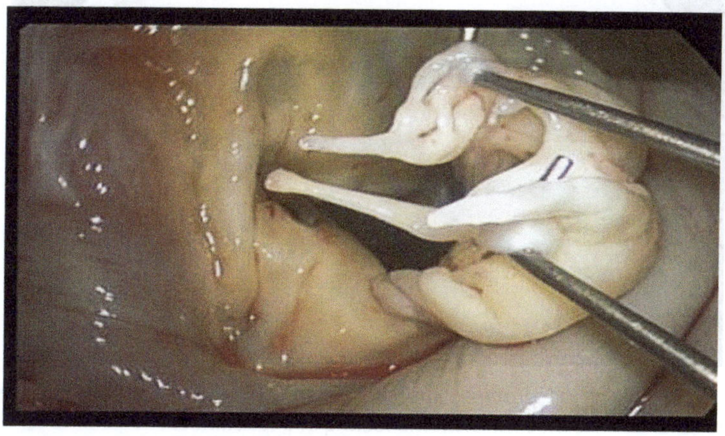

Fig. 5.4: Examination of the leaflets with two hooks. The elongation is used to define the prolaptic area. Segment A1 serves in most cases as a reference point.

The quadrangular resection is the typical repair technique for a single local prolapse of a posterior segment. It is necessary to define the width of the prolapse exactly.

Cutting out of the prolapse

Then, with the furthermore spread out prolapse, one can mark the area to be cut out. With the long knife a short incision is made at the base in the middle part of the area about 1 mm above the ring. The same has to be done right and left 2 mm inside of the known prolapse limits (▶Fig. 5.7). Now the extension of the resection area is defined and with the slightly curved scissor the excision with a cut from incision to incision is performed.

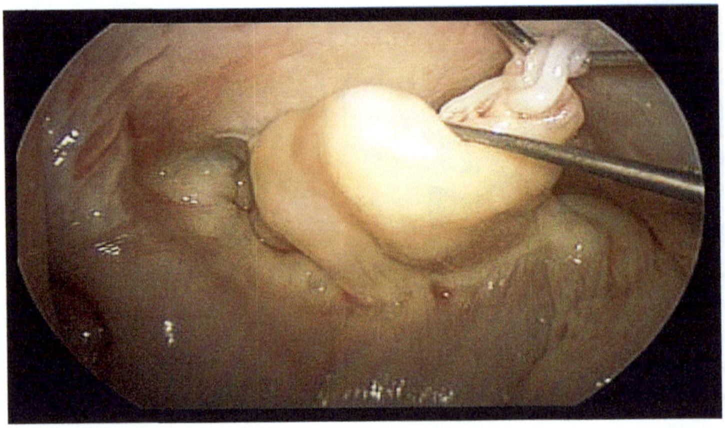

Fig. 5.5: The prolaptic area is spread out by using a nerve hook and lifted up in the middle part.

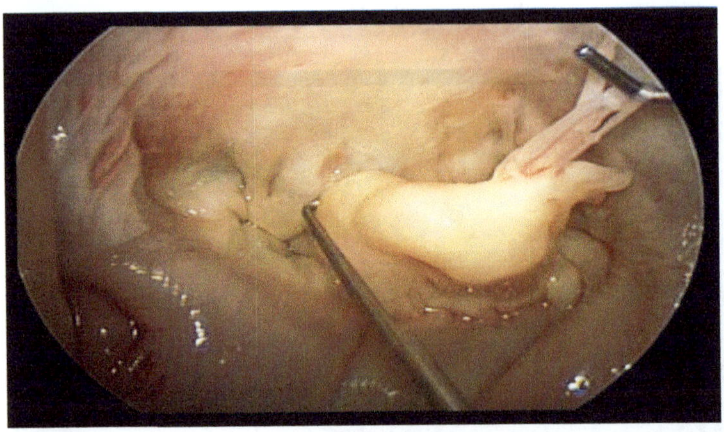

Fig. 5.6: Definition of the prolapse limits by two hooks. One spreads out the prolapse whereas the other defines the limit with the feeling of a resistance.

Then the situation has to be checked again using the hooks. It must be clear that all of the supernumerary tissue was cut out and sufficient tissue was left for closing the gap. At this moment a necessary correction of the cutting edges is possible. Sometimes if too much tissue was cut out, the technique must change from a relatively simple direct closure of the gap to a more complicated technique of a sliding plastic. It would be wrong to try and close the gap with too little tissue because of the resulting tension in the leaflet. Here the high risk of a postoperative rupture remains.

After cutting out the prolapse, enough tissue should remain for closing the gap.

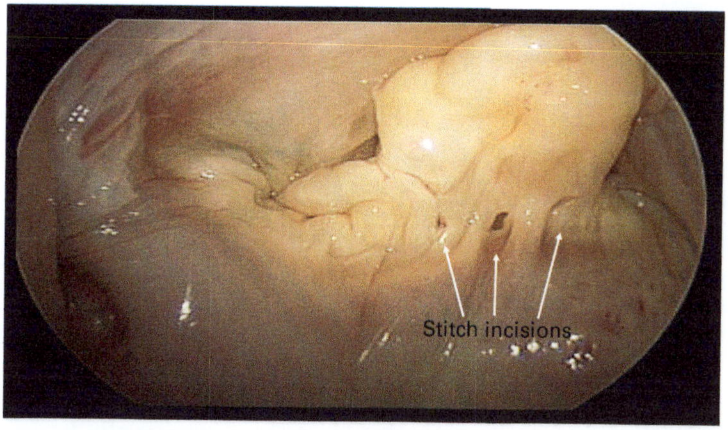

Fig. 5.7: Stitch incisions mark the cutting edges for escision of the prolaptic leaflet part.

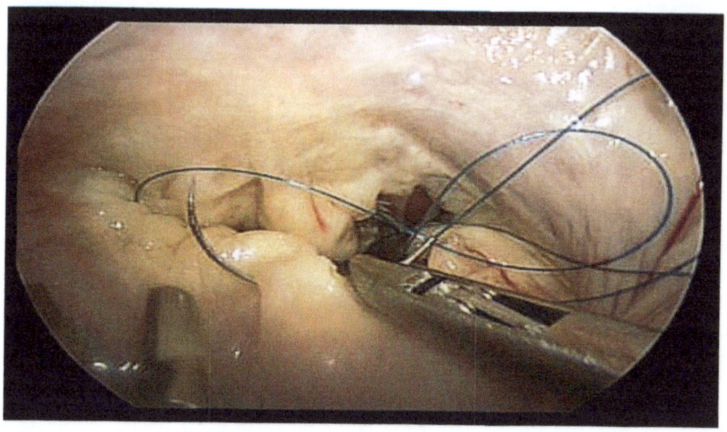

Fig. 5.8: For narrowing of the native ring, the first stitch leads from atrium to ventricle and the second comes back on the other side of the gap.

Narrowing of the annulus

If the process of cutting out is satisfactory, the suture for narrowing the native ring follows. With a 3–0 Cardionyl® suture the first stitch starts about 2 mm next to the limit of the removed area from atrial to ventricular direction through the annulus and comes back complementary on the other side (▶Fig. 5.8).

Now a narrowing of these parts of the annulus results if the two ends of the suture are pulled up with a forceps (▶Fig. 5.9). In the next step it is easy to make one or two more stitches through the more atrial ring parts. When the suture is tied into a knot a smaller posterior circumference will result and the two edges of the leaflet come together (▶Fig. 5.10).

It is absolutely necessary to avoid an annulus that is too small with too much narrowing. That may lead to a complete change in the architecture of the posterior ventricular wall at this area with the possibility of decreasing the blood flow through the circumflex artery or resulting even in mitral valve stenosis.

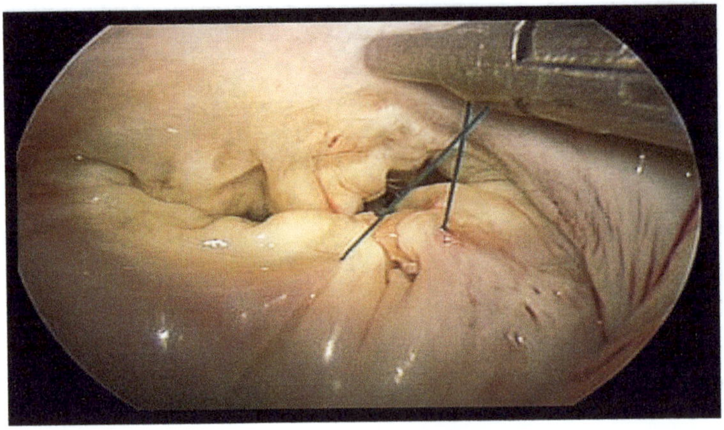

Fig. 5.9: The ring is narrowed by using a forceps to pull up the two ends of the suture.

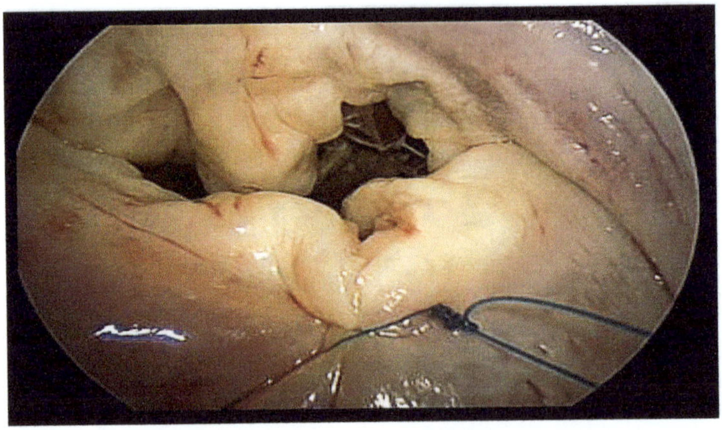

Fig. 5.10: With a second stitch the fixation of the ring parts is finished, and after the knot is tied a perfect narrowing of the ring results.

> Avoid narrowing the native annulus too much. The result would be a small orifice area of the valve (cave mitral valve stenosis!) and/or a decreased function of the circumflex artery.

Closure of the gap

After that procedure a closure of the remaining two parts of the posterior leaflet is normally easy. In principle, two different techniques are in use. One is the closure with single sutures and the second is a double running suture.

The use of single sutures is a more complicated technique because repeated knots have to be placed. The advantage could be a safer situation in case a suture ruptures. The resulting gap will be limited by the remaining sutures and will produce a small regurgitation only. A running suture is easier to handle but could lead to a complete gap with a high-grade regurgitation. The choice between these two options depends on the quality of valve tissue, the surgeon, and personal experience.

For both techniques it is important to make the single stitches very carefully and exactly. It seems not to make a difference if the suture starts at the free edge or at the level of the native annulus. But for orientation, and to be sure that the two free ends of the leaflet meet exactly, it may be advantageous to start at the free edge.

From a practical point of view the suture starts at the right side of the gap at the outermost point of the free edge. With a hook this point should be identified exactly and should be lifted up (▶Fig. 5.11). Then the first stitch can be carried out under a clear view and controlled conditions. With the needle inside, the free edge can be kept in position with the needle holder. Then the hook can change to the left side of the gap and the opposite point for the first stitch can be identified (▶Fig. 5.12).

After bringing the two instruments closer together a second stitch can be placed. Replace the hook with a forceps to remove the needle. Then the knots may be tied and the second suture for a single-suture process or the first of a running suture can be made.

For the use of a running suture the safety of the gap closure can be increased by carrying out a double running suture with both ends. It takes a bit more time but at the end a more stable situation for the leaflet is reached, and two ends for tying the knots after finishing the suture are available.

If there is enough tissue it seems to be advantageous to use a more inverting technique instead of a simple suture of the cutting edges. This leads to a smoother surface of the posterior leaflet with little thrombotic potency. The inverted technique may be performed with an in-and-out stitch at the same side of the leaflet part at both sides of the gap. Then the smooth surface of the leaflet parts comes together and a very nice result is often reached (▶Fig. 5.13).

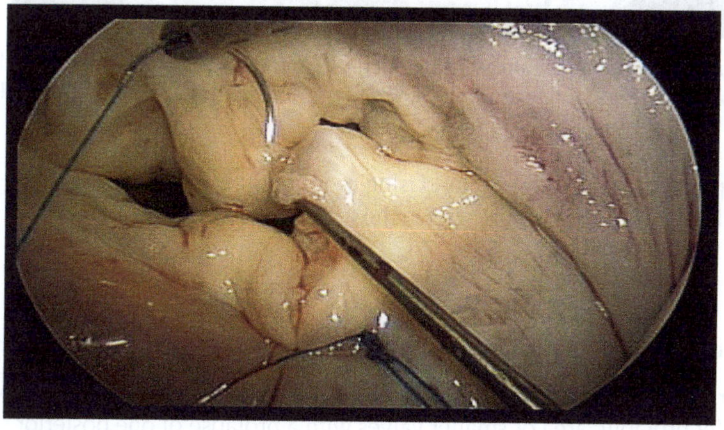

Fig. 5.11: With a hook the rest of the leaflet will be lifted up before the first stitch is performed.

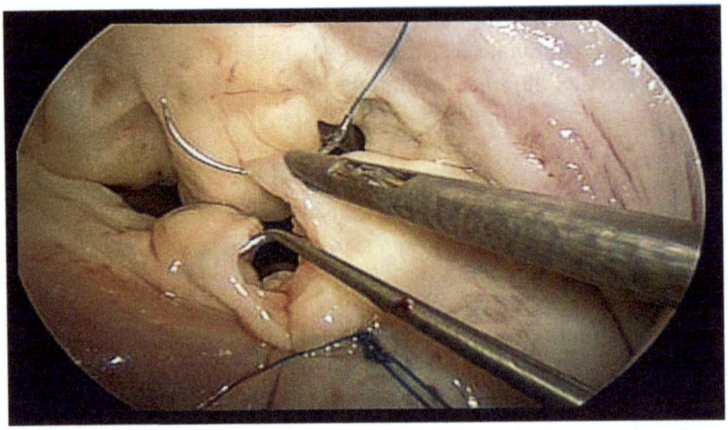

Fig. 5.12: After performing the first stitch the needle keeps the tissue in a lift-up-position and the hook changes to the other side of the gap.

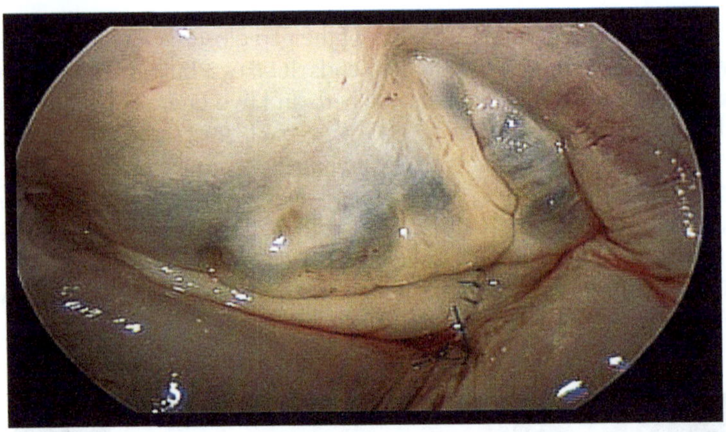

Fig. 5.13: An excellent result after cutting out a prolapse in P2 and reattaching the left leaflet parts with an inverting stitch technique. A "smiling" of the mitral valve can already be seen.

> The gap has to be closed exactly. Using a double running suture leads to a safe and stable closure without any gap in the leaflet tissue.

5.2 Triangular resection

In comparison to the quadrangular resection the triangular resection is more often used for a smaller prolaptic area or smaller valves with a prolapse of one posterior segment.

5.2.1 Pathological anatomy

Typically the prolapse has a rather triangular shape with the tip at the native ring and the base at the free edge (▶Fig. 5.14). Very often the reason for this type of prolapse is a

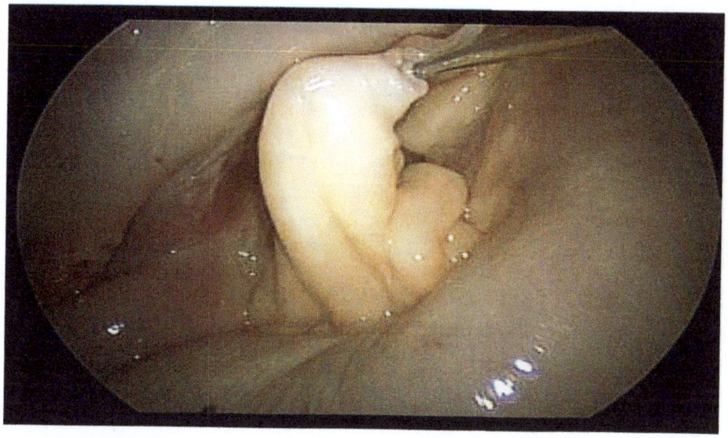

Fig. 5.14: A typical finding of a more triangular prolapse with the tip at the ring and the prolapse at the free edge.

ruptured primary chord. Here a very localized expansion of the leaflet tissue follows and so the typical triangular shape develops. In some cases the function of secondary chords at this area is completely preserved. Here the problem may be solved with the insertion of a neochord alone.

5.2.2 Theoretical remarks

In contrast to quadrangular resection a smaller part of the leaflet will be resected. The cutting line follows the triangular shape of the prolapse and the right and left line meets about 2 mm before the annulus is reached. So an additional narrowing of the native annulus is avoided and the original circumference is still preserved.

> The typical prolapse for a triangular resection is smaller than for quadrangular resection and never includes more than one segment. A narrowing of the annulus is normally not necessary.

5.2.3 Practical realization

Identifying the prolapse

The main steps for an explicit definition of the prolapse are the same as described for quadrangular resection. In contrast to this procedure here it is often enough to take a hook and to spread out the prolapse with a tension at the area of the ruptured chord (▶Fig. 5.15). Then it is very easy to see how the adjacent normal parts of the leaflet stay in a normal position and because of that are curved down.

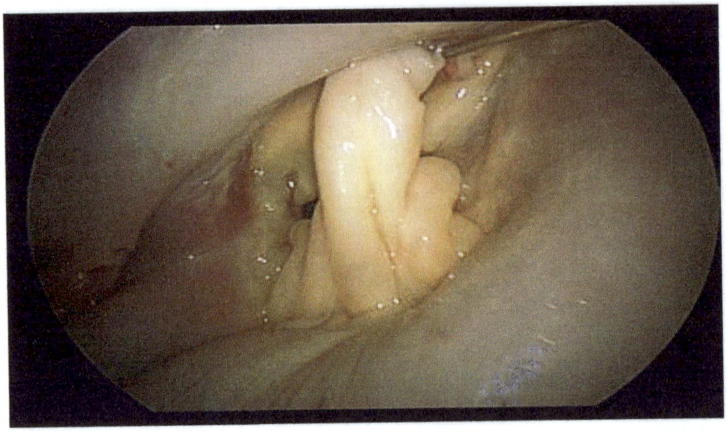

Fig. 5.15: A ruptured chord as a typical reason for a triangular prolapse. It is simple to show the prolapse and the normal tissue with one hook.

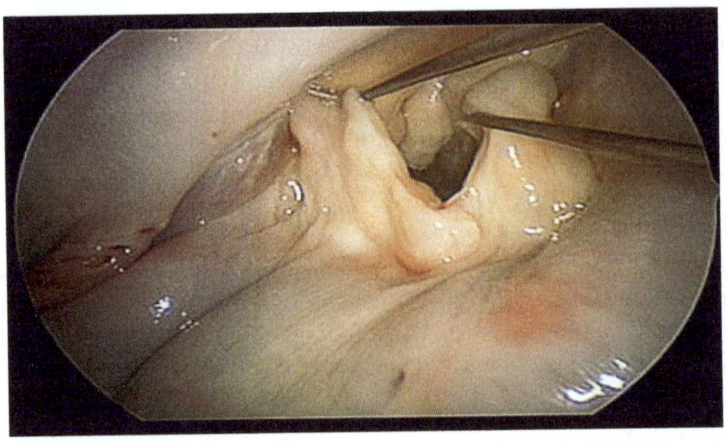

Fig. 5.16: With the scissor the prolaptic tissue is cut out from the free edge to the native ring.

Cutting out the prolapse

If, one time, the prolapse is spread out with one hook, a small incision at the tip of the triangle (near the annulus!) can be made. This is not a basic condition for cutting out, but it helps for orientation and avoids a cut that is too deep.

With the slightly curved scissor, the cuts are directed from the free edge to the annulus (or even to the existing incision). It starts only a few millimeters besides the middle of the prolapse (where the hook should be placed) and goes to the ring under excision of a triangular piece of leaflet tissue (▶Fig. 5.16).

Narrowing of the annulus

In cases of a triangular resection as described, a narrowing of the annulus is not necessary. Normally the remaining leaflet parts allow a direct and tensionless closure. If the gap is too large against the original plan the narrowing of the ring has to be performed as described in Section 5.1.

Closure of the gap

The procedure of closing the gap is exactly the same as described in Section 5.1. Therefore, refer to that section for more details.

After triangular resection of the prolapse, a simple closure of the remaining gap is enough. Because of the small diseased area, a very stable result can be achieved.

5.3 Sliding technique

Especially in mitral valve diseases with very large prolapses and a large height of the posterior leaflet, the sliding plastic may help reach an optimal functional result with a normal anatomy of the valve. In contrast to the techniques with resection of leaflet tissue alone, the remaining leaflet tissue will be used here for closing a large defect at the basic of the leaflet without any annulus compression in most cases.

5.3.1 Pathological anatomy

Two different groups of mitral valve diseases can be identified for using the sliding plastic. The first is a group with too much tissue all over at the posterior part of the valve (and often also at the anterior part). The main problem of Barlow's disease, described in literature, is often the height of the posterior leaflet with more than 20 or 25 mm (▶Fig. 5.17). Therefore, the resection with a direct closure of the gap only leads to SAM phenomena. It results in a shifting of the coaptation area more to the anterior leaflet

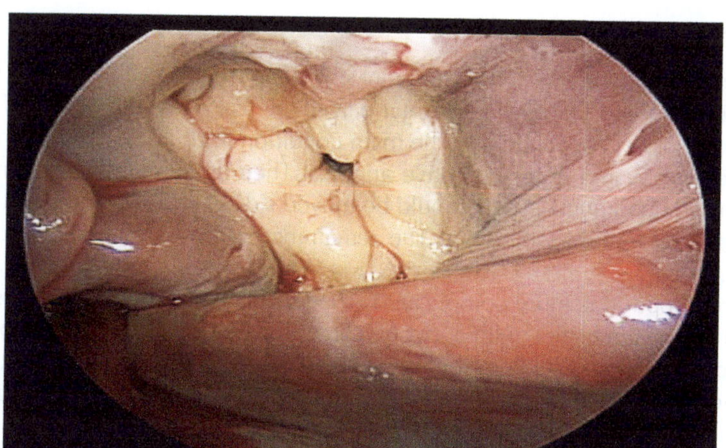

Fig. 5.17: So-called Barlow's disease is characterized by much tissue especially in the posterior leaflet area.

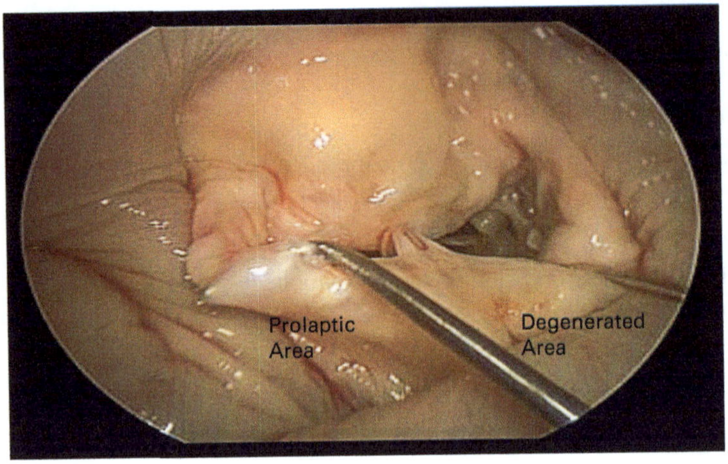

Fig. 5.18: A restricted leaflet area may lead to prolaptic adjacent tissue.

and deeper in the left ventricle. The consequence is often a systolic narrowing of the left ventricular outflow tract.

The second group is a mitral valve disease that includes degenerated prolaptic parts of the posterior leaflet. Sometimes the degeneration of one part may lead to an excessive stress of adjacent tissue parts with the development of a prolapse beside the degeneration (▶Fig. 5.18). The sliding plastic may help rebuild the degenerated leaflet part using the adjacent prolaptic parts of the leaflet.

The sliding plastic shows the best results in two groups of mitral valve diseases: the so-called Barlow's disease, with too much tissue in many parts of the valve, and the coexistence of a degenerated part beside a prolaptic part of a leaflet.

5.3.2 Theoretical remarks

From a geometric point of view two different situations are imaginable. One is the complete shifting of a mobilized quadrangular part of the leaflet after resection of an adjacent prolaptic or degenerated part. The main condition to do that is to detach the part that is intended to shift from the native annulus. Then the annulus will be narrowed and the solved quadrangular part should be moved sideways and re-fixed at the annulus ("quadrangular sliding plastic"). The remaining cutting edges may be closed as described.

The second option is more complicated. The typical situation for using this is a degenerated part of the leaflet (with a low height) followed by a prolaptic part on the left or right side that is too high. For rebuilding the leaflet, and to receive a perfect shape, it may be advantageous not to remove the prolaptic part but, rather, the degenerated part. Then the remaining prolaptic part may tip over sideways into the gap, and the former lateral border of the prolaptic part will be the new edge for fixation at the native ring when the remaining gap is large. The former free edge of this part becomes the new edge (as a cutting edge after quadrangular resection) for closing the gap ("tip sliding plastic"). This procedure might have an advantage because a narrowing of the annulus is often not necessary and a continuous normal height of the posterior leaflet results.

5.3.3 Practical realization

Identifying the diseased parts

As in the theoretical remarks described, two different diseased parts of the posterior leaflet should be identified. With two hooks the complete posterior leaflet is spread out step by step.

For a quadrangular sliding plastic, a degenerated part can be identified by hooks. A clearly reduced mobility of a part of the posterior leaflet will be seen. For this part it is not possible to move the leaflet into the left atrium and chords that are too short can be felt (▶Fig. 5.19).

All other parts of the posterior leaflet seem to be in an acceptable functional situation. For making a decision it should be clear that the expansion of the degenerated part should not exceed 2 cm in order to avoid a too small valve diameter after annulus compression. That means a switch of the technique on the other side if the degenerated parts are larger.

For the tip sliding plastic a point will be found in a typical situation where one hook shows very reduced leaflet mobility and the other spreads out a prolapse (▶Fig. 5.20). Then, with two hooks the complete diseased part should be defined and every part should be determined. The ideal situation would show a degenerated part with an extension such as the height of the prolaptic part (▶Fig. 5.21). When this correspondence is given the variability for using this technique is higher than for a quadrangular sliding plastic because it will prevent any annulus from narrowing.

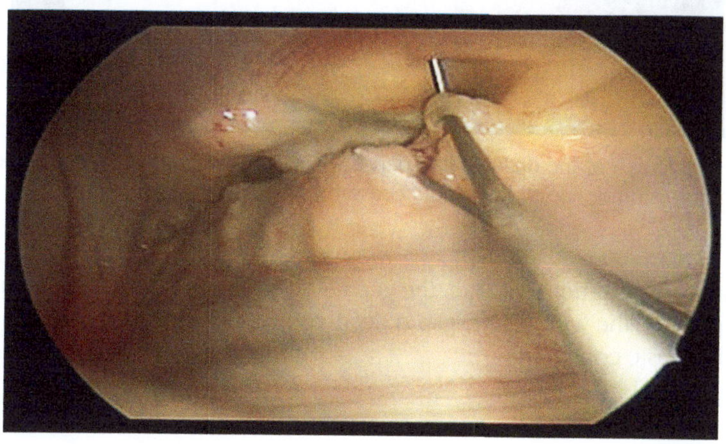

Fig. 5.19: In cases of degenerated leaflet parts the posterior leaflet cannot be moved into the atrium.

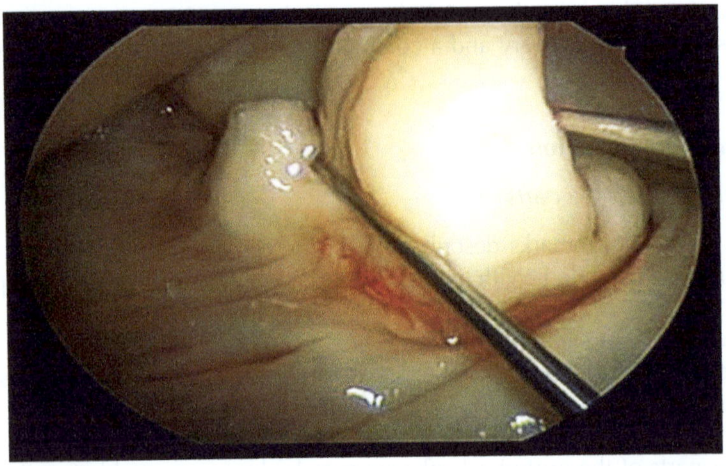

Fig. 5.20: Demonstration of both important points for a tip sliding plastic. One part of the leaflet is degenerated (left hook) whereas the other one is prolaptic.

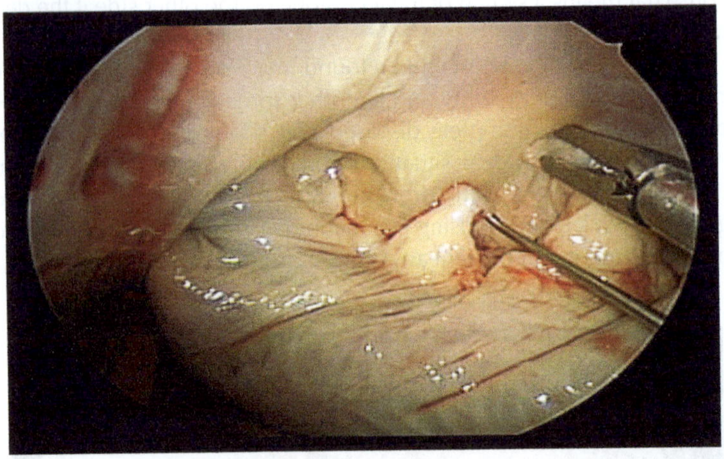

Fig. 5.21: The length of the degenerated part is equal to the height of the prolaptic part. An annulus compression or narrowing is not necessary.

For a successfully sliding plastic, the geometric relations between the remaining leaflet part and the width of the gap is decisive. A clear demonstration of all main points is a basic condition.

Cutting out of diseased part(s)

After identifying the degenerated part the chords of this area may be lifted up with a hook. With the knife or a more curved scissor the chords are cut (▶Fig. 5.22). It should be clear that with every chord cut the area of the degenerated part that has to be

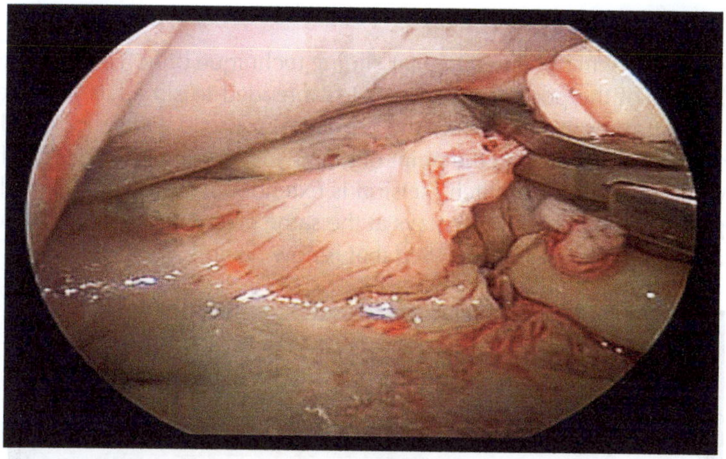

Fig. 5.22: After identifying the degenerated part the chords of this area should be cut out.

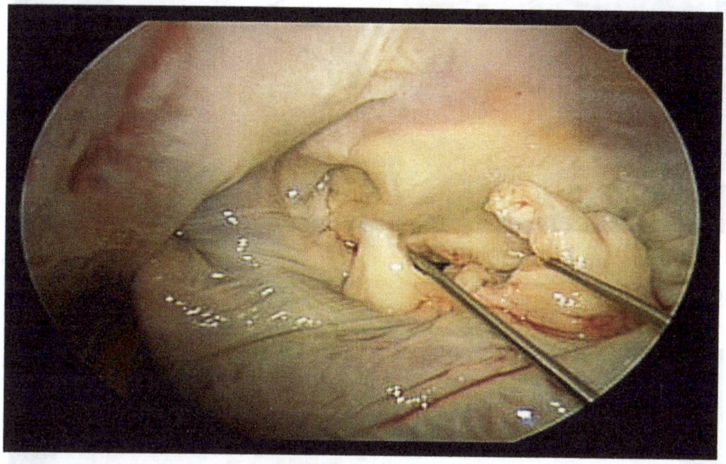

Fig. 5.23: Cutting out the diseased area after chords are cut. With a hook, the limit of the area is lifted up and should be cut until the native annulus is reached.

removed will grow. In the following step, with two hooks the mobilized but diseased area will be defined again.

Next to one hook the first limitation (right or left) is spread out and with the curved scissor the leaflet is cut directly beside the hook until the annulus is reached (▶Fig. 5.23). At the other limitation it should be performed accordingly. Then the degenerated part is removed between these two incisions with a complete detachment from the annulus.

After this procedure, a gap results that has a limitation of two normal leaflet parts or one normal leaflet part and a prolaptic part. This difference determines the next steps and the technique that has to be used for closing the gap.

Retiring the leaflet

This step is necessary in the quadrangular sliding technique only. To be able to narrow the ring, the part of the posterior leaflet that is intended to slide has to retire directly above the annulus. For this procedure the free edge is spread with a hook and with the knife a short incision is made at the point of the needed width (▶Fig. 5.24). Then, with the slightly curved scissor the stitch incision is extended parallel to the annulus to the cutting edge (▶Fig. 5.25). The hook stays at the same position as before. At the end, an about rectangular leaflet area is achieved that is now flexible.

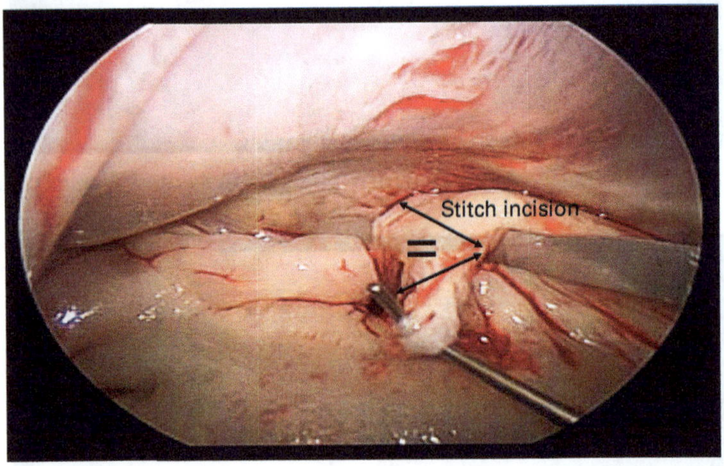

Fig. 5.24: The right point for the stitch incision is the height of the prolaptic tissue that is equal to the width of the gap.

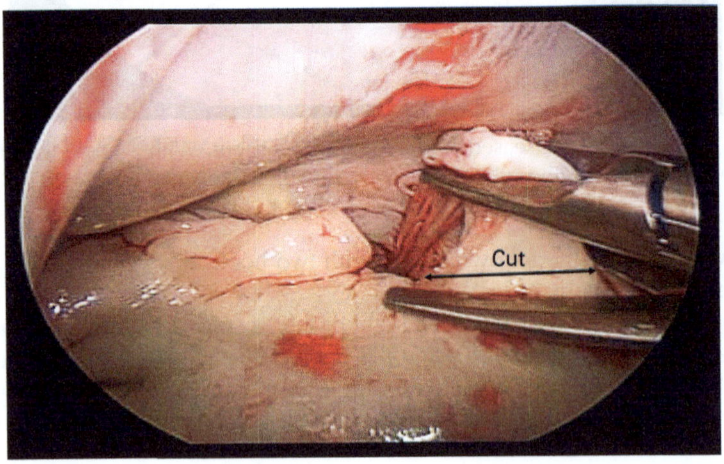

Fig. 5.25: After performing the stitch incision the leaflet part has to be cut off from the native annulus in the direction of the cutting edge.

For a quadrangular sliding plastic an adapted part of the (normal) leaflet has to be retired. This step is necessary for this type of plastic only.

Narrowing of the annulus

A narrowing of the annulus is necessary for closing the gap only in cases of two remaining leaflet parts with the same and normal height. It is absolutely important to be sure that the remaining distance of the gap is small enough to allow a tension-free adaptation of the leaflet parts. Otherwise the primary result may be satisfactory but after some days a rupture of the leaflet probably will lead to a new regurgitation.

In cases with one prolaptic part of the leaflet the ring has to be narrowed only when the distance of the gap is larger than the height of the prolaptic leaflet part that is planned for "tip sliding plastic." It is important to know that the narrowing distance of the annulus should be kept as small as possible to avoid a stenotic component of the result.

The narrowing of the annulus follows the same rules as described for quadrangular resection. It is not necessary in cases with tip sliding plastic.

Under compliance of all of these ideas the narrowing of the annulus is the same procedure as already described (for details see Section 5.1).

Sliding and refixation

This procedure is one of the most important parts of the complete sliding plastic. In the end there is no difference in the technique used for both types of sliding. The logical steps are the closure of the gap at first and the re-fixation of the moved leaflet part for finishing the procedure.

For closing the gap a 4–0 Cardionyl® suture should be used. With a hook the free corner of the quadrangular sliding area or a point about two thirds of the height of the prolaptic leaflet part should be found and then the tissue has to be lifted up (▶Fig. 5.26). Then the first stitch goes through that point. The hook can be removed and the next stitch with the same suture goes through the annulus where the limitation of the opposite leaflet ends. Next it might be advantageous to make some knots to fix this point while the ends of the suture should be kept at the same length (▶Fig. 5.27).

With this step the gap was closed at the basic. Now it is relatively easy to use one end of the suture to make a running suture from the basic to the free edge of the leaflet. The length is defined in quadrangular sliding with the height of the moved leaflet part. For tip sliding plastic the next stitch should not be done when the tissue comes under tension (▶Fig. 5.28).

In the end the re-fixation of the folded leaflet parts follows. For that the remaining end of the suture can be used (▶Fig. 5.29). As alternative procedure and for more safety both ends of the first suture will be used for closing the gap as a double running suture. With an additional suture the folded leaflet part can be fixed at the annulus double.

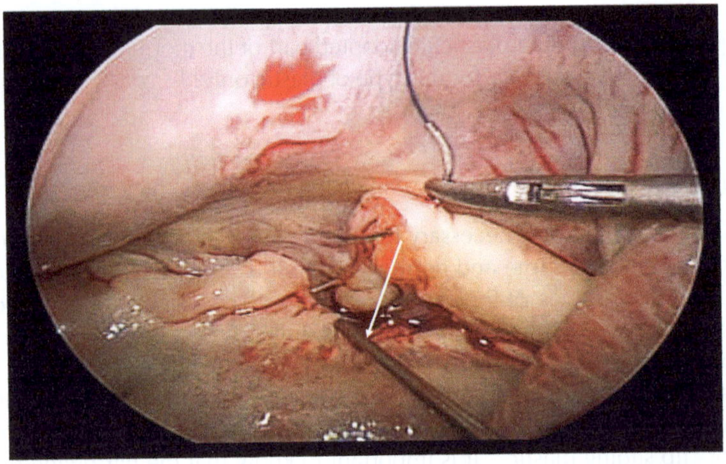

Fig. 5.26: With a hook, the point for the first stitch will be found. Normally it is the free corner of the sliding tissue or, even in cases of prolaptic tissue, a point that is about the height of two-thirds of the leaflet height.

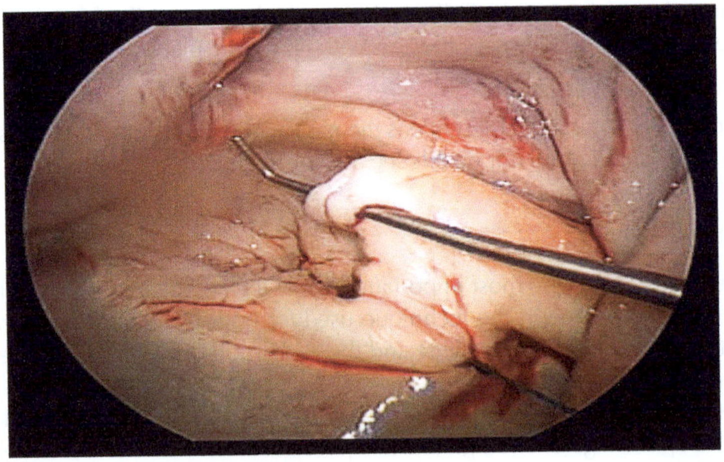

Fig. 5.27: The first stitches are made and the suture is tied. A running suture to the free edge should then follow.

5.4 Neochords – preformed loops

The technique of Neochord implantation using preformed loops was first described by Ulrich van Oppeln and Friedrich Mohr. It was the first time that we had a standardized technique for the replacement of ruptured chords using the minimally invasive technique. It was a special pleasure for me to learn it from these two pioneers of endoscopic mitral valve surgery.

One of the main characteristics of preformed loops is the fixed length in combination with a defined part for the fixation at the papillary muscle (▶Fig. 5.30). A special situation can be found when more than one loop is preformed but the fixation part is the same (loops in groups of two or three for one fixation at the papillary muscle).

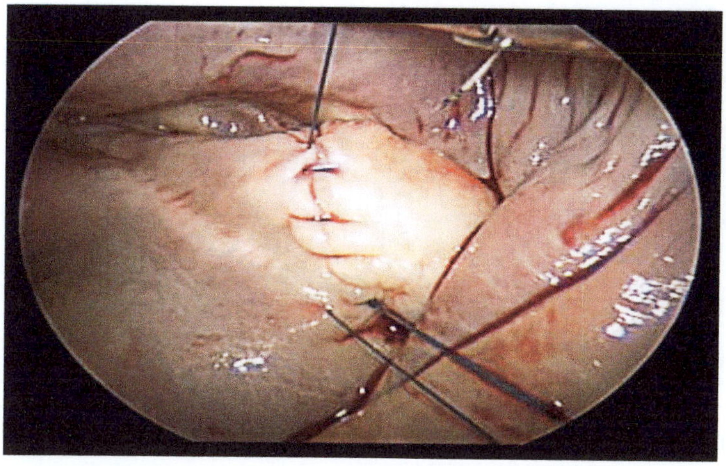

Fig. 5.28: The height of the leaflet is defined by the height of the sliding tissue or, even in tip sliding plastic, as long as the suture can be made without higher tissue tension.

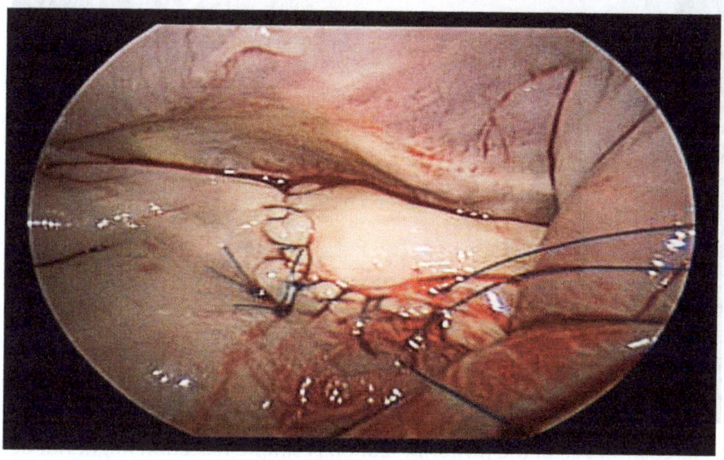

Fig. 5.29: After sliding, the leaflet tissue has to be fixed at the native ring with the other end of the suture.

5.4.1 Pathological anatomy

One main finding for using Neochords is one or more ruptured chord(s) with a large prolapse of the posterior leaflet. It is relatively easy to show these findings. In many cases the prolapse includes more than one segment. This means that the area is larger than can be repaired with either a simple excision or a sliding plastic alone (▶Fig. 5.31). After a typical reduction of the prolaptic area with a quadrangular or triangular resection, the resulting leaflet shows, furthermore, not enough stability or a more prolaptic situation. Additional support seems to be necessary.

A different situation might be found for the anterior leaflet. Here, a ruptured chord often cannot be found. The typical findings are elongated chords. As a consequence a prolapse can be seen but it is not clearly defined as in a posterior leaflet (▶Fig. 5.32).

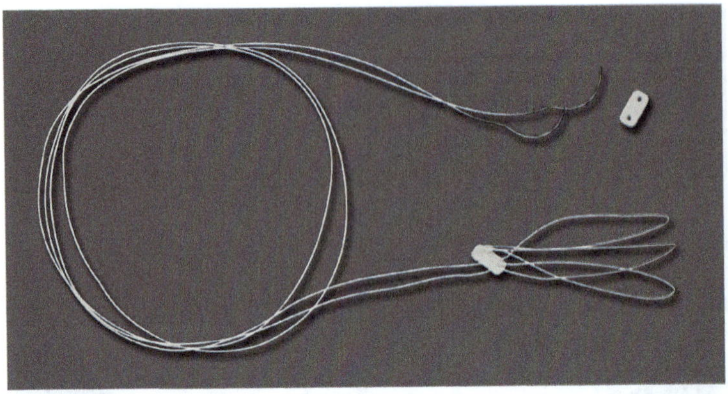

Fig. 5.30: Typical preformed loop (single loop) made from a Gore-Tex® suture. The pledget marks the transition between fixed length and the defined part for fixation.

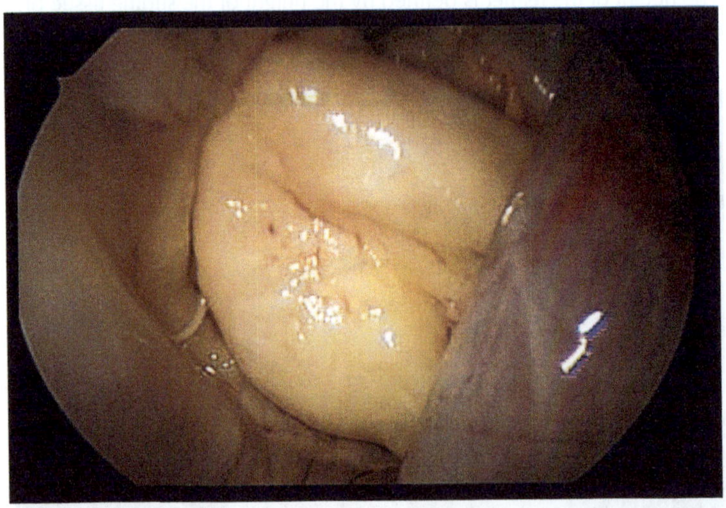

Fig. 5.31: A large prolapse of the posterior leaflet. A simple resection might not be enough to reach a long-term stable result.

But in some cases a ruptured chord also can be the reason for regurgitation. A large and clearly defined prolapse can be found here (▶Fig. 5.33). Another problem is the impossibility of cutting out parts of the anterior leaflet because of the missing coaptation area after that.

The typical finding for the use of Neochords is a prolapse of the anterior leaflet or a larger area of the posterior one. Preformed multi-loops allow connecting several points of the free edge with one papillary muscle.

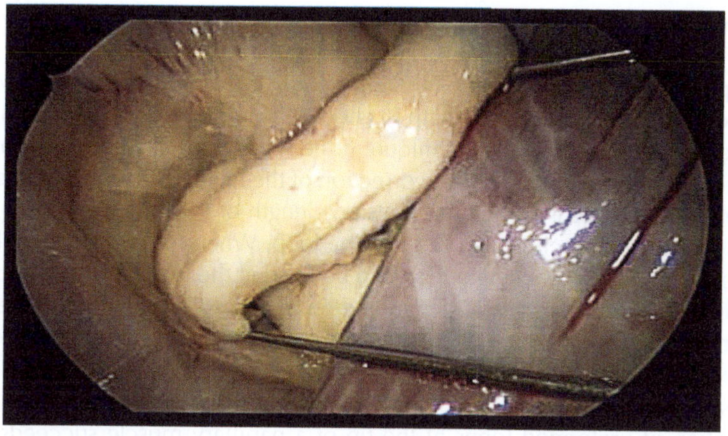

Fig. 5.32: Typical prolapse of the anterior leaflet. A ruptured chord is rare but elongated chords are often seen. The definition of the prolaptic area is more difficult in these cases as in posterior prolapses.

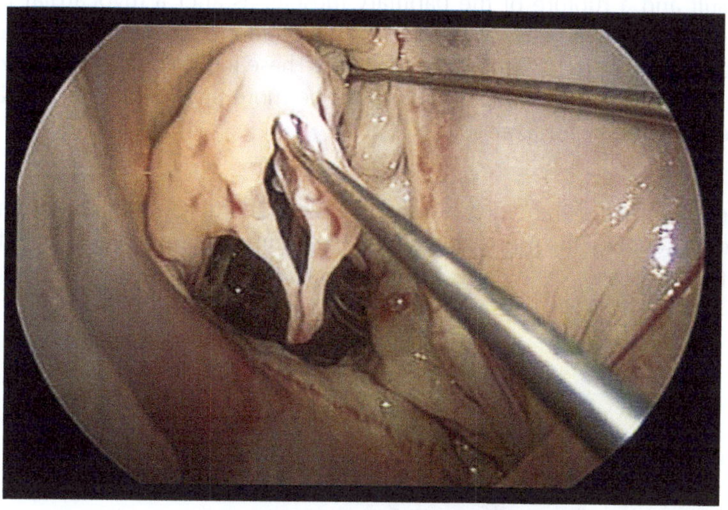

Fig. 5.33: In the case of a ruptured chord of the anterior leaflet the prolapse is clearly defined.

5.4.2 Theoretical remarks

There are three prerequisites for implanting Neochords. First, a suture will be needed, the thrombogenic potential of which is as low as possible. Second, the length of the Neochord has to be defined exactly. And third, the suture has to be safely anchored at both sides: the papillary muscle and the leaflet.

It has gained acceptance to use sutures made of Gore Tex® for implanting Neochords. These sutures are very smooth in a combination with high durability and strength. But because of these characteristics a safe implantation needs a special suture technique that will be described further on (see Section 5.4.3).

To define the exact length of the chords an instrument for measurement was developed by Friedrich Mohr (▶Fig. 5.34). This instrument helps especially when the technique of preformed loops is used. Although handling this instrument is easy it needs some experience to find the right length to choose the right preformed loop. This shows one of the disadvantages of this technique. If the length is defined and the preformed loop is fixed at the papillary muscle a correction of the length is no longer possible.

Another disadvantage is sometimes the same length of the bundle of loops in a preformed Neochord that includes more than one loop. When fixed at the papillary muscle it saves time when every single loop can be fixed at the leaflet with a simple suture (for details see Section 5.4.3). But depending on the anatomical situation the distance between the papillary muscle and the free edge of the leaflet is different for every single loop especially when the tip of the muscle is more lateral and the ruptured chords are numerous.

The fixation of preformed loops at the tip of a papillary muscle succeeds with the pledget-supported basic part of the preformed Neochord. A general aspect is to respect that the fixation has to be done in the more fibrous part (i.e. at the tip) and not with sutures through the muscle tissue (▶Fig. 5.35). After incorrect placement of sutures necrosis can result and a rupture of the papillary muscle, as after a myocardial infarction, could be seen after some days. The loops of the preformed Neochord will be fixed at the free edge of the muscle with Prolene sutures. These junctions are normally very stable. Only in cases with an endocarditis can it be more problematic to find a durable area of the leaflet tissue for fixation.

> The measurement of the exact distance between the tip of the papillary muscle and the free edge of the (normal) leaflet is the main condition for a successful use of this technique.

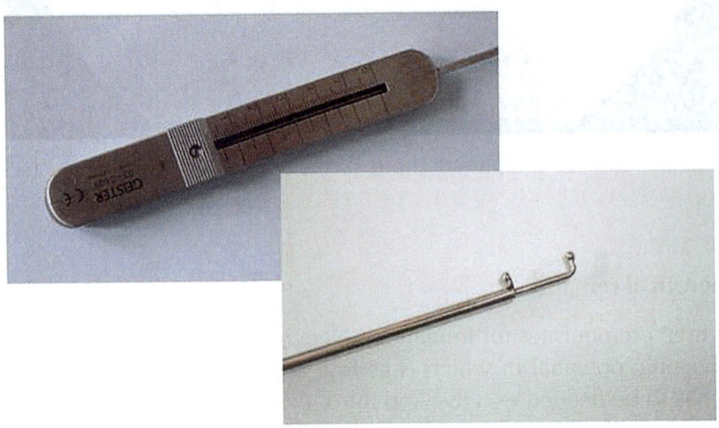

Fig. 5.34: An instrument to measure the length between the tip of a papillary muscle and the free edge of a leaflet (developed by Fred Mohr).

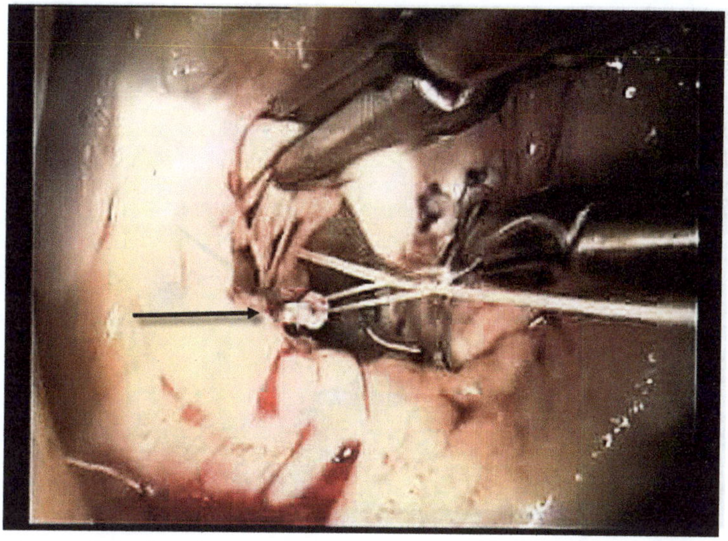

Fig. 5.35: The preformed loop has to be fixed at the fibrous tip of a papillary muscle (as every Neochord, arrow).

5.4.3 Practical realization

Identifying the diseased parts

For the use of Neochords the definition of diseased parts means primarily to define these areas of the leaflets that show an abnormal mobility in direction to the left atrial cavity. It seems to be very helpful to find an area that shows normal mobility for using this area as a reference point (often it is the area A1). In order to define normal mobility it should be clear that the line of coaptation is about 2 mm above the free edge, and this line should be found at the level of the annulus or a bit underneath in the direction to the ventricle (▶Fig. 5.36). So all other segments can be compared with this reference point and it can be shown which area needs a new chord. Especially if there is a prolapse at an anterior segment, a clear definition of the exact point for reinsertion of a Neochord can be found.

For carrying out the procedure it is only necessary to use two hooks. One hook should stabilize the reference point and with the other hook all other segments are controlled systematically. In the end it will quickly be clear where abnormal mobility was detected and a new chord is necessary. As a rule and at minimum one new chord per prolapsed segment should be calculated.

Measurement of the chordae length

The length between the tip of the papillary muscle and the free edge of the leaflet is the distance for the loop. For defining, two things will be needed: a reference point and an instrument for measurement.

The reference point is found in many cases by the fact that with one hook a seemingly normal part (in many cases segment A1) is spread. Then, with the instrument introduced by Mohr, the length between the tip of the papillary muscle and the reference

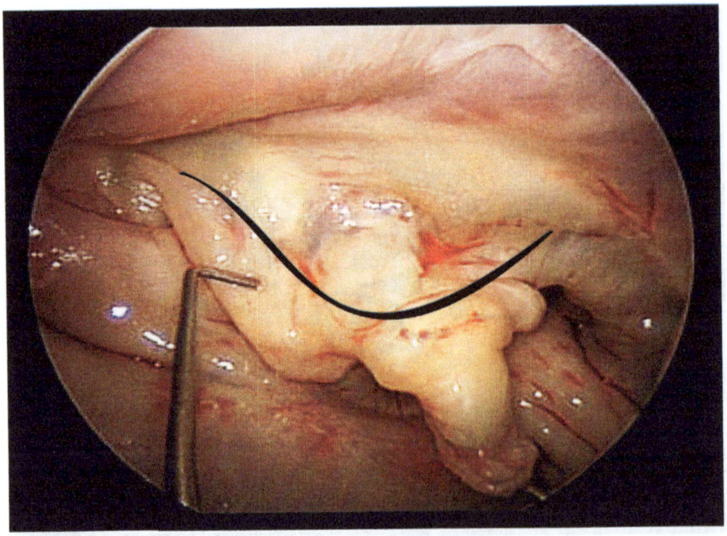

Fig. 5.36: Definition of the coaptation line with a hook and pulling back the leaflet part. This is basic for measuring the right length of the Neochord.

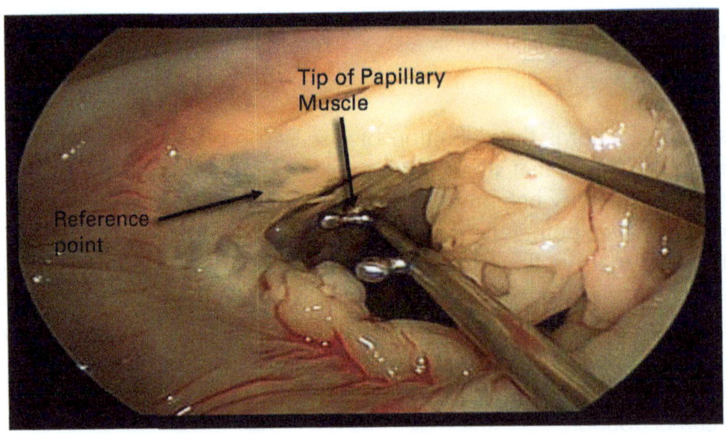

Fig. 5.37: After definition of the reference point the distance between the tip of a papillary muscle and the free edge can be measured using the instrument.

point is measured (▶Fig. 5.37). The only problem is that sometimes the difference in length between the tip of the papillary muscle and the reverence point and the tip of the papillary muscle and the segment that needs a new chord is different. For these cases the measurement should be made between the planned implantation point at the tip of the papillary muscle and the level of imaginary closure line of the mitral valve.

A larger prolapse has to be brought more into the left ventricle than a smaller one. This different degree of correction shows the other disadvantage of the measurement for chordae with fixed lengths. The different distances between the insertion point of a new chord at the free edge of a segment and the tip of the papillary muscle makes it more difficult to define the correct length in these cases. The more the free edge has to

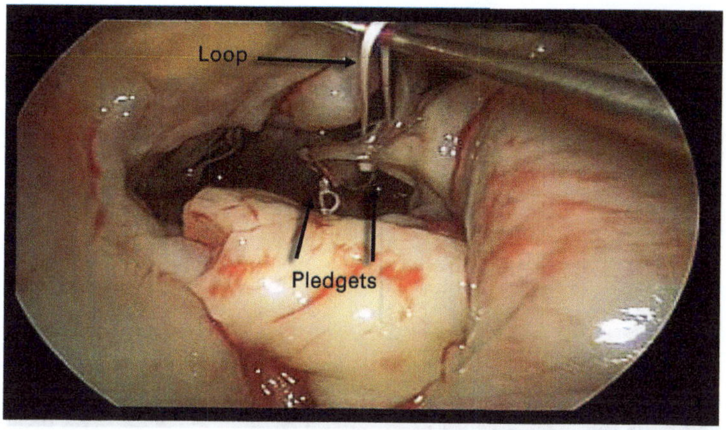

Fig. 5.38: After stitching the ends of the preformed loop through the tip of the papillary muscle, knots should be tied over a secondary pledget (see the left of the pledgets).

shift into the left ventricle the more the coaptation line moves to the middle of the leaflet. This leads to an additional influence on the correct length of an artificial chord and makes measurement difficult.

For an exact measurement the definition of diseased area and the closure line is necessary. Different distances need different lengths of Neochords.

Implantation of preformed loops

The implantation technique of preformed loops follows two steps: the first is the fixation of the loop at the papillary muscle. The second is the junction between the loop and the free edge of the leaflet.

The fixation of the loop at the tip of the papillary muscle succeeds with both free ends of the suture. There are two facts that have to be respected: the suture should go through the fibrous part at the tip of the muscle, and before a knot is tied a second pledget should be used for better support of the knots (▶Fig. 5.38).

After fixation of the loop at the papillary muscle and as last step every single loop has to be brought in a stable junction with the predefined area of the leaflet. This will be carried out using a Cardionyl® suture for every single loop. After the needle was led through the loop the stitch has to go through the free edge of the leaflet underneath the coaptation line. For better orientation the fixation point often can be defined by the area where the rest of the original primary chords will be found (▶Fig. 5.39).

5.5 Neochords – flexible length

The use of Neochords with flexible length is a newer technology and is based on the idea of an individual shifting of the free edge of the leaflet. Because of that it is also called the "gliding edge technique."

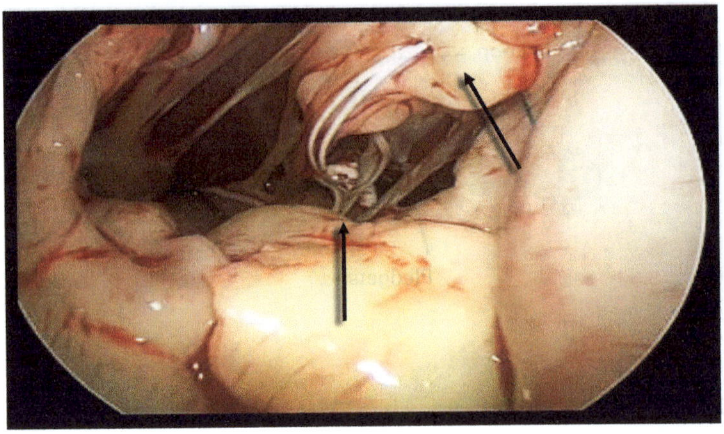

Fig. 5.39: The single loop has to be fixed at the free edge of the leaflet to achieve a stable junction between the papillary muscle and the prolaptic leaflet area (arrows).

The main idea is to use a Gore Tex® suture for the junction between the papillary muscle and the free edge of the leaflet without any predefined distances or lengths. As a consequence it is more function-oriented working with the ability to change the situation as long as the best result is probably reached.

5.5.1 Pathological anatomy

The findings for the use of Neochords with a flexible length are the same as described in Section 5.4.

5.5.2 Theoretical remarks

For using Neochords with a flexible length the same prerequisites apply as for preformed loops. However, in contrast to the method for preformed loops the definition of a length and a special instrument for measurement is not needed.

All decisions for the Neochord implantation will be made while the procedure is carried out and the only orientation is the functional result. This means that in cases of more than one implanted chord the differences in length and the choice of papillary muscles for fixation can differ substantially.

A fixation of the suture at the tip of the papillary muscle with pledgets and knots will also not be needed. Because of using a simple loop that follows a double stitch to fix the suture at the fibrotic part of the muscle tip, an ischemic injury is scarcely to be expected. In every diastolic situation the suture is under no stress, and therefore the loop at the muscle tip allows tissue perfusion for a short time. Besides these ideas it seems to be simple to perform a double stitch without knots in comparison to the necessity to make knots in the depth of the left ventricle. Especially for endoscopic surgery with small incisions it can make the difference for a better handling.

The functional orientation described in the paragraph before includes the ability to move the free edge not only in a direction from the atrium to the ventricle alone but also in the opposite direction. From that, the main advantage of the technique results are described here: the ability to correct the movement of the free edge and the length of the Neochord in both directions as long as the seemingly best result is achieved. For practical use this means that regardless of reference points or the widening and shape of the prolapse, the leaflet can be corrected with enough coaptation area and enough flexibility for the different filling situations of the left ventricle.

It is clear that the danger of overcorrecting has to be respected. Therefore the result (water filling test) should be tested with more than a normal filling situation. For practical use more than 150 ml water should be used to test the functional result. If an overcorrection is made after the first 100 ml no leakage will be seen, but after a filling of 150 or 200 ml the leaflet will be pulled back into the left ventricle and a leak will be seen.

Using the gliding edge technique allows adapting the distance between the papillary muscle and free edge more functionally. Measurement is not necessary.

5.5.3 Practical realization

Identifying the diseased parts

Refer to Section 4.4 for information on identifying diseased parts.

Measurement of the chorda length

In contrast to preformed loops, an exact measurement of the length of the loops is not necessary. The reason is the only functional orientation of the length with the possibility to change the position of the free edge of a prolapsed segment as long as it seems to be needed. Therefore, the length of the chords follows the functional result and it does not matter how long the Neochords are in the end. The ability to let the free edge glide up and down causes the lower rates of failing for Neochord implantation procedures.

Implantation of flexible chords

The implantation follows three steps: suturing the tip of papillary muscle, suturing the free edge of the leaflet, and fixation after correct positioning of the free edge.

For suturing the tip of the papillary muscle the anterior leaflet should be lifted up with a forceps or a hook to see the muscle tip. Now with a forceps the tip may be fixed and the first stitch can be made (▶Fig. 5.40). It is absolutely necessary to make the stitches through the fibrotic part of the muscle tip and to make the stitches deep enough (with enough tissue in the loop at the end). Now the suture may be pulled through to create two halves of the complete suture. This can be done with the needle holder alone while the forceps keeps the tip. It is simple to repeat the procedure a second time to create the loop.

Then, two ends of the suture result at the outside with a loop through and around the tip of a papillary muscle. If more than one loop is necessary a small clamp can keep the first suture and a second or third one may be carried out. It seems to be simpler to create all loops with stitches through the tips of the papillary muscles at first. Then the suturing of the free edge should follow.

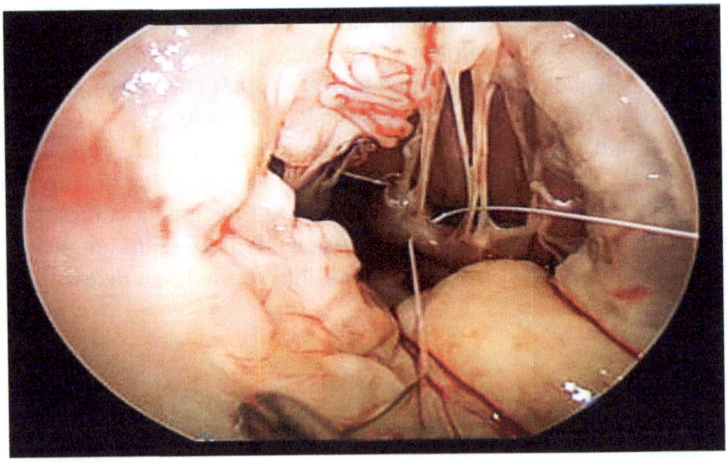

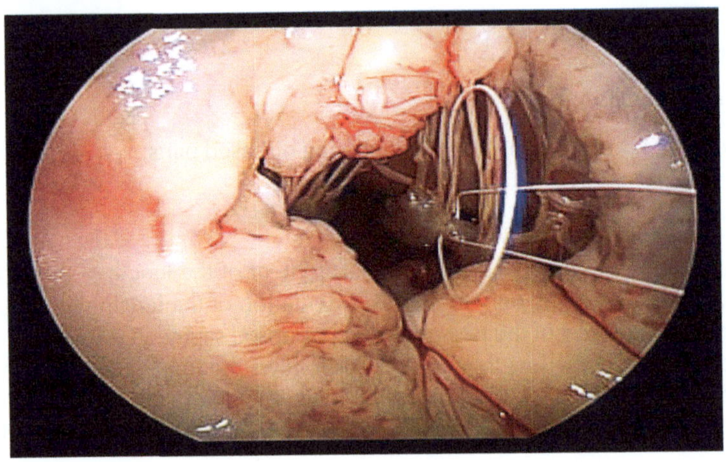

Fig. 5.40: For the first stitch the tip of the papillary muscle should be lifted up using a forceps to pull up the chords of this muscle. The rest of a ruptured chord is clearly seen. To take this photo the videoscope was more pushed in than when working on the leaflets.

> The first step when using this technique is suturing the Gore Tex suture through the tip of the papillary muscle. The fibrotic part must be used.

The right position for the sutures that go through the free edge will be found by using a hook and pulling back the leaflet tissue. With every end of a suture a double stitch has to be performed through the free edge. After every second stitch the needle should lead through the loop of the thread to get a single knot (▶Fig. 5.41). This procedure has to be repeated for every suture, which should result in a Neochord at the end (i.e. for every suture that goes through the tip of a papillary muscle). Respect the fact that measurement or estimation of the length is not necessary.

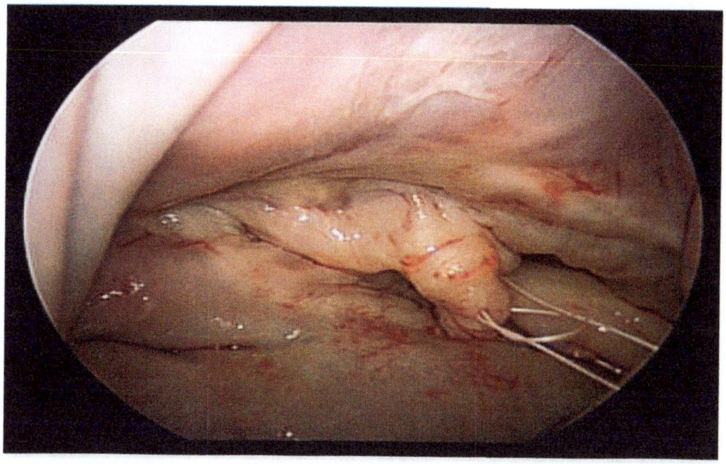

Fig. 5.41: Every end of the suture will be stitched through the free edge of the leaflet twice. The second stitch should lead through the loop of the thread and result in a simple knot.

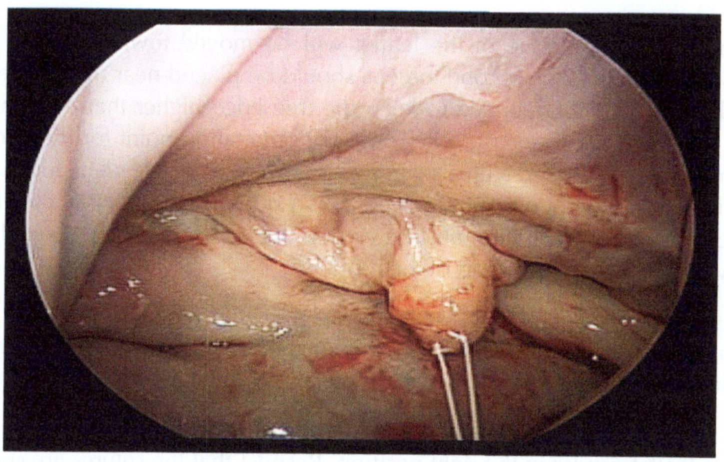

Fig. 5.42: Typical situation after performing all stitches before the free edge should be moved.

When the suture ends are stitched through the free edge a single loop should be created. Additional knots, especially in the depth of the left ventricle, should be avoided.

Then, all sutures create a loop through the tip of a papillary muscle and both ends of all sutures create a loop with a single knot through the free edge of the leaflet (▶Fig. 5.42).

But the prolapse is still not corrected; this last step is simple indeed. With one forceps the two ends of the Neochord will be fixed about 5 mm above the leaflet, and with a

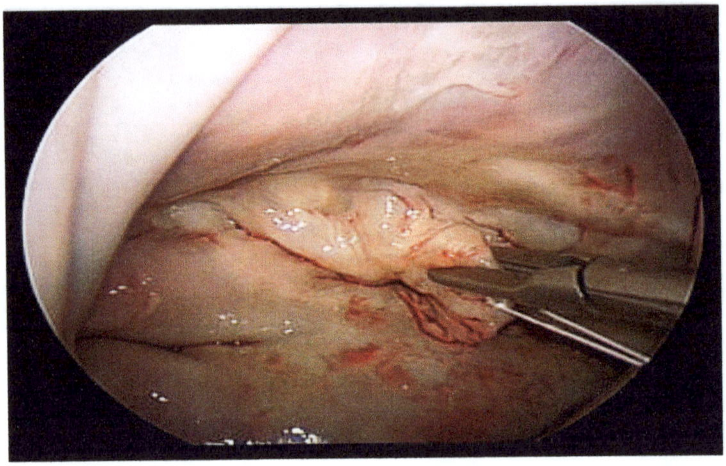

Fig. 5.43: For leaflet movement, one forceps keeps the two ends of the suture (not shown in the photo) while the other moves the free edge up and down.

second forceps the free edge of the leaflet will be moved toward the left ventricle (▶Fig. 5.43). To do this, the second forceps should be placed near the simple knots of the Neochord. It is recommended to keep the free edge higher than too deep at the end. It is not necessary to measure it. The main orientation point for the widening of movement is the comparison with a seemingly normal part of a leaflet. However, this is not so much a question of one millimeter as it is a question of the individual morphology of the valve. This procedure must be carried out with every single Neochord, that is, with every single supported part of the prolapse.

> The correction of the prolapse follows moving the free edge with two forceps. The position of the free edge should be estimated only. Further corrections are possible.

Now the leaflet can be in the right position. Respect that the sutures are still in position and the ends are outside the thorax. A functional water test that is filled into the left ventricle shows the functional result. If leakage is seen when the first 100 ml are filled in the free edge it should be moved toward the left ventricle at this point. However, if leakage is developed after 150 or 200 ml, an overcorrection may be done and the free edge should be pulled back 1–2 mm. To do that, the two forcepses are needed again but the first one now fixes the Neochord underneath the leaflet and the second pulls back the free edge. Then the water test should be repeated. This procedure can be repeated as long as necessary to achieve a perfect functional result (▶Fig. 5.44).

> Using the water test the functional result can be assessed. If further correction is necessary the free edge can be moved up and down until the final knots are tied.

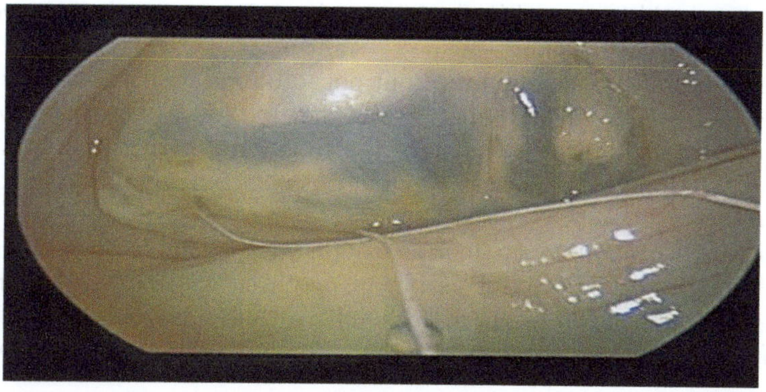

Fig. 5.44: The leaflet was moved in the optimal position and the water test shows an optimal functional result. The ends of the suture remain untied until the best result is reached.

5.6 Artificial rings

5.6.1 Theoretical remarks

The implantation of artificial mitral rings is a basic technology in mitral valve repair. Whether there is a necessity to implant an artificial ring in every case is one of the most discussed issues in mitral valve surgery. The more artificial rings on the market the more the different advantages and disadvantages are discussed. This discussion will not take place in this book. For further information, refer to special literature or product prognosis.

There is no doubt that the use of artificial rings leads to two effects: the stabilization of the mitral valve system after repair and/or to a narrowing of the native annulus in cases of annulus dilatation.

The main goal of mitral valve reconstruction is the plastic repair of a clearly defined structural valve injury. In these cases – and they should be most cases – the result after repair should lead to a nearly normal function and the artificial ring should have a supporting function only.

From this point of view the type of artificial ring used might depend on the type of reconstruction. In cases of quadrangular resection of the posterior leaflet and a narrowing of the posterior part of the annulus, a more stable artificial ring (rigid or semi-rigid) should be used. However, in cases of Neochord implantation only, and without changes to the native annulus, a more flexible ring could be a good choice.

The question cannot be answered here as to whether an artificial ring is necessary. In many cases mitral valve disease is not a local problem of one segment or one ruptured chord. However, this disease concerns the whole mitral valve system. The consequence of this point of view is to accept that the main problem (which leads to the indication for the operation) has to be solved with a reconstruction. However, in the end the complete valve needs support. If one accepts these ideas it is not a question of whether a ring is necessary but of which ring should be used for which situation.

Rigid rings are characterized by a relatively stiff core that keeps the ring in shape and allows supporting a mitral valve very effectively. In both situations with a dilated ring or a normal ring with structural leaflet injuries these rings may help preserve a good functional result over a long time.

Alternatively, these rings often turn out not to be the best solution for patients with a high tension at the posterior leaflet that follows a dilated left ventricle. Here, sutures can often be torn out of the tissue and then the ring is without function. A solution could be more flexible rings, such as semi-rigid or complete flexible rings.

Regardless of the ring used, an anticoagulation therapy will be needed in the early follow-up period. In patients with sinus rhythm, prophylactic therapy with Warfarin® or an analog drug is enough for two or three months. After this time the endothelialization of the artificial ring has developed and the risk for thromboembolism is very low.

Artificial rings should be used in most cases. The preferred model depends on the anatomical situation, personal experiences, and technical conditions.

5.6.2 Implantation technique

For implantation of artificial rings, the same rules apply as for open heart surgery. This means, respect the anatomical course of the circumflex artery or avoid an injury of the non-coronary cusp of the aortic valve. In the end, the individual technique for ring implantation may be used as in open heart surgery. The only issue that has to be respected is the careful use of the knot pusher to avoid knots without fixing the ring ("air knots"). Especially at the area of the anterolateral commissure, special attention should be paid because the direction of the knot pusher movement changes here (▶Fig. 5.45).

Another main point is the correct placement of sutures. Not only is localization concerned but also, primarily, depth. A safe placement with enough tissue is absolutely necessary for a long-lasting stabilization effect of the artificial ring. Especially at the area between 2:00 and 7:00 it may sometimes be difficult to see the correct

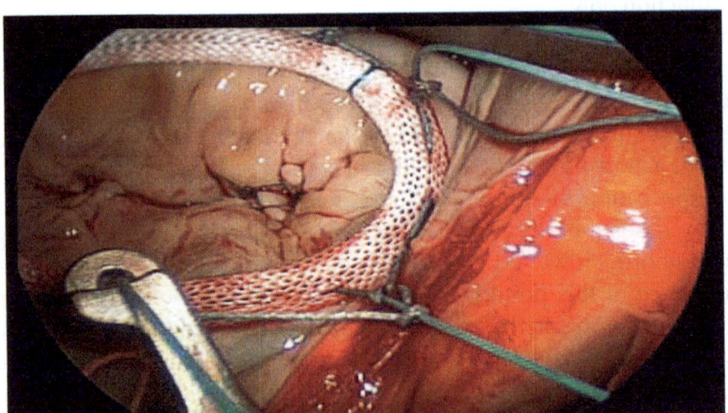

Fig. 5.45: Using the knot pusher at the area between 02.00 and 04.00 clockwise means to change the direction of the knot pusher movement to reach exact knots.

localization and to stitch the needle deep enough. Here some tricks may help, such as the multifunctional use of instruments (for details see Section 6.4).

For better handling it seems to be advantageous to place all sutures at first inside and arrange them step by step around the thoracic incision on the outside (▶Fig. 5.46). Now the ring may be fixed with a clamp directly in front of the surgeon and the sutures that are placed at the anterior part of the native annulus may stitch through the artificial ring in succession (▶Fig. 5.47). After that, the clamp can be removed and the assistant should hold the ring and the last sutures can be stitched through (▶Fig. 5.48).

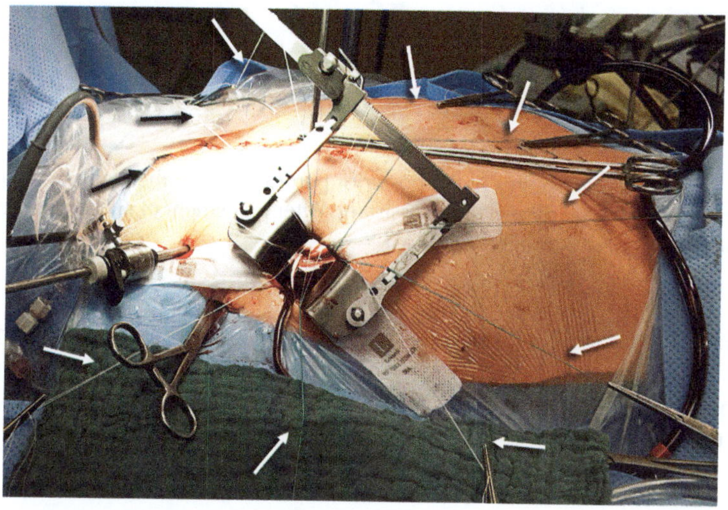

Fig. 5.46: All sutures for ring implantation are placed and arranged on the outside.

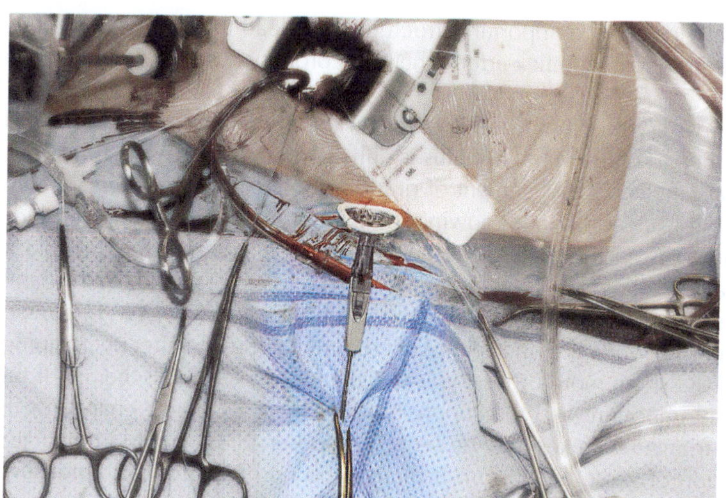

Fig. 5.47: The artificial ring will be kept by a clamp in front of the surgeon, and suture placement starts with the sutures of the anterior part of the ring.

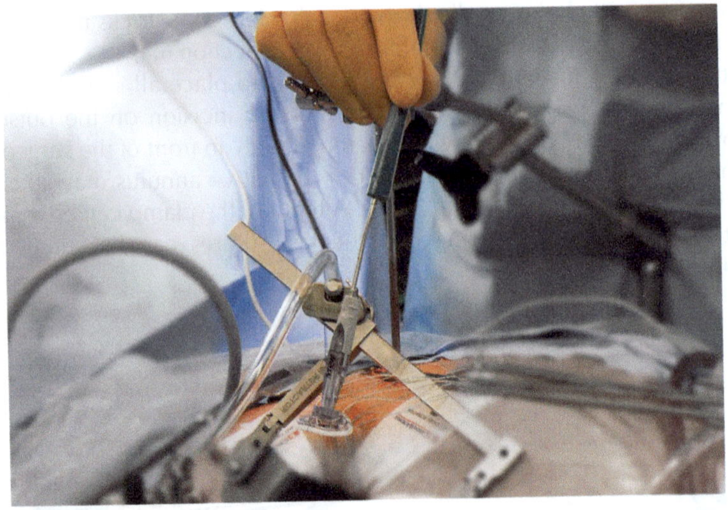

Fig. 5.48: For placing the sutures at the posterior part of the ring, the clamp will be released and the ring holder will be moved to the assistant. After placement of all sutures the ring may be brought in and the sutures may be tied.

> The implantation technique of artificial rings follows the same rules as in open heart surgery. In cases with a downsized annulus pledget supported sutures can prevent subsequent detachment of the artificial ring in the posterior part of the annulus.

5.6.3 Complications

Anatomical closeness to important structures may lead to three main opportunities for complications: the circumflex artery, the non-coronary cusp of the aortic valve, and the AV node.

It is no mystery that the distance between the circumflex artery on the outside and the posterior part of the mitral annulus is only 3–4 mm (▶Fig. 5.49).

Therefore, the correct placement of ring sutures is particular necessary between 6:00 and 10:00. It is clear that not knowing the left coronary angiogram is an indispensable prerequisite to assess the anatomical situation. Then, either the sutures are placed directly into the native ring or about 3–4 mm more in the left atrium parallel to the native ring.

There is no sign if a suture encloses the circumflex artery or seals this vessel because of tissue tension while the ring is implanted. Only at the end after declamping the aorta does the ECG show more or less typical signs for myocardial ischemia. If the artery is functionally important and the supply area is large, a massive change of the normal ECG with triangular spikes may be seen. This observation should immediately lead to the suspicion of vessel occlusion. If there is no normalization within a few minutes, one should no longer wait for a correction of suture placements in the critical area.

It is not necessary to use cardioplegic solution again. After fibrillation of the heart the left atrium may be reopened. Because of a suspected vessel occlusion only and

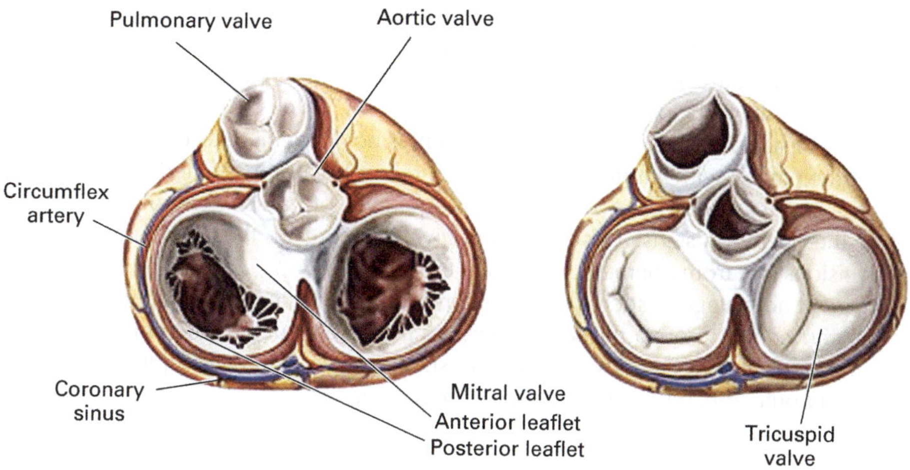

Fig. 5.49: Anatomical structures around the native mitral ring cause an opportunity for complications.

uncertainty about which suture causes the occlusion, all sutures between 6:00 and 10:00 have to be removed and replaced elsewhere.

The second possibility for a complication is to catch the non-coronary cusp of the aortic valve with a suture in the middle of the anterior part of the ring. This leads to aortic regurgitation that may be seen in the TEE at the end of the procedure under physiological circulatory conditions. Sometimes an immovable cusp may be seen. If the regurgitation is new in comparison to the aortic valve function before the operation was started, no other reason should be expected for that. The only way out is to reopen the left atrium after fibrillation of the heart and remove the sutures from the middle anterior ring area. Of course new sutures have to be placed.

The last complication, and in respect to frequency of occurrence the fewest, is the development of an AV block. This may be registered at the end of the procedure but it has no consequences at this time. Only if the AV block exists longer than three or four days might a pacemaker implantation be necessary.

Complications after implantation of an artificial ring in most cases result from an injury to the circumflex artery. Careful and very exact placement of sutures helps avoid this.

5.7 Emergency exit

5.7.1 Theoretical remarks

When endoscopic surgery starts, and also any time after starting, all efforts to repair a mitral valve can fail. The typical situation is a time-consuming reconstruction using many different techniques with the result that the way was wrong. In transesophageal echocardiographic examination, a higher regurgitation has to be registered. This is the right time to make a decision for the purposes of the patient. It has to be internalized absolutely that valve replacement is much better than a bad reconstruction result. In other words: the surgeon's intention to be proved right cannot outweigh a good functional result for the patient.

If these ideas are accepted, valve replacement is not longer a disaster. It is one option to treat the patient with a mitral valve failure if reconstruction has failed. Everybody involved – the team, the cardiologist, and the patient, of course – should realize this before the operation starts. This agreement gives the surgeon the opportunity to make the decisions free from nonmedical ideas at the right time.

The great advantage of such a development during surgery is that valve replacement can be carried out through the same access as the reconstruction attempt. This means that all advantages of an endoscopic access, such as lower traumatic injury and a better pulmonary outcome, will be preserved for the patient.

5.7.2 Practical performing

If there is a situation after a failed reconstruction it is clear that all implanted sutures and the artificial ring have to be explanted if valve replacement has to be carried out. After that, a part of the anterior leaflet may be resected to get enough space for the valve. With the knife, a small incision near the annulus is made at the anterior leaflet about 2 mm beside the anterolateral commissure (▶Fig. 5.50). Then, with the curved scissor, the anterior leaflet can be separated from the annulus until the posteromedial commissure is nearly reached (▶Fig. 5.51). To preserve the function of chords the main part of the anterior leaflet should be completely resected along the free edge. In the end, a 2 mm band with leaved primary chords can be included into the sutures for valve replacement very simply (▶Fig. 5.52). The posterior leaflet usually should be leaved completely.

Then the sutures for valve replacement should be implanted. It has become apparent that in many cases a larger needle is advantageous to a smaller one. It is important that the gliding characteristics of the sutures used are as good as for ring implantation. This

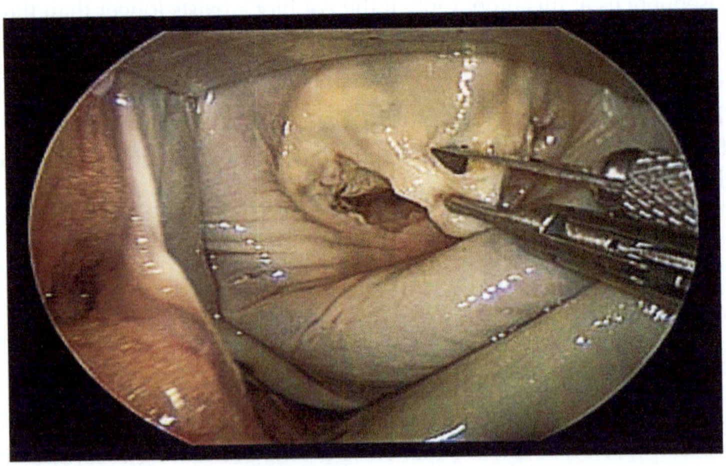

Fig. 5.50: To cut out a part of the anterior leaflet, a stitch incision near a commissure should be performed.

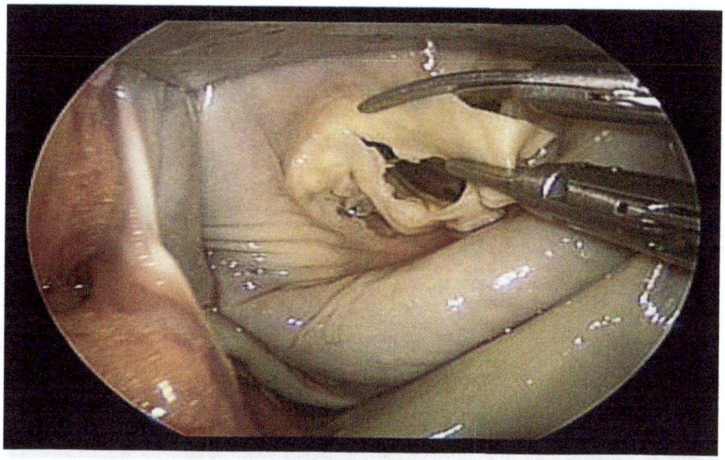

Fig. 5.51: With the more curved scissor the anterior leaflet will be released from the anterior native ring.

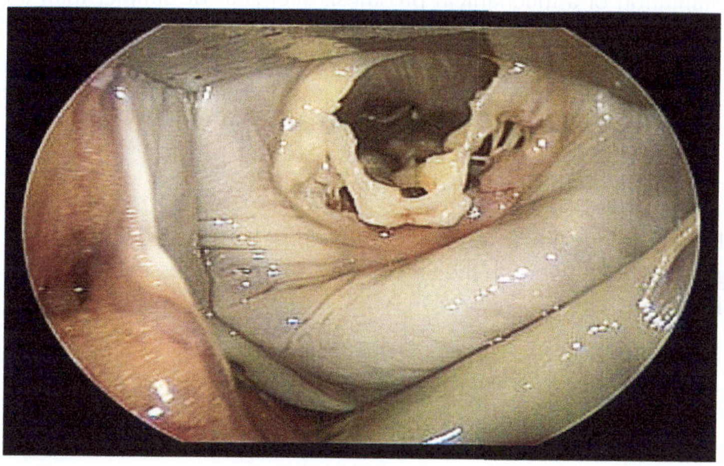

Fig. 5.52: For preservation of ventricular function a small band with main chords (first chords) should remain inside. They may be involved in the sutures for fixing the valve.

helps avoid trouble with knots that do not exactly reach the right position and could cause in paraprothesis leakage. Because of the different function, this problem is more important for valve than for ring implantation.

Using the videoscopic technique it is simple to verify the positioning of the sutures. As in open heart surgery, the structures around should be respected.

> Replacement of the mitral valve using an endoscopic technique is not a complicated procedure. Chords should remain as they are.

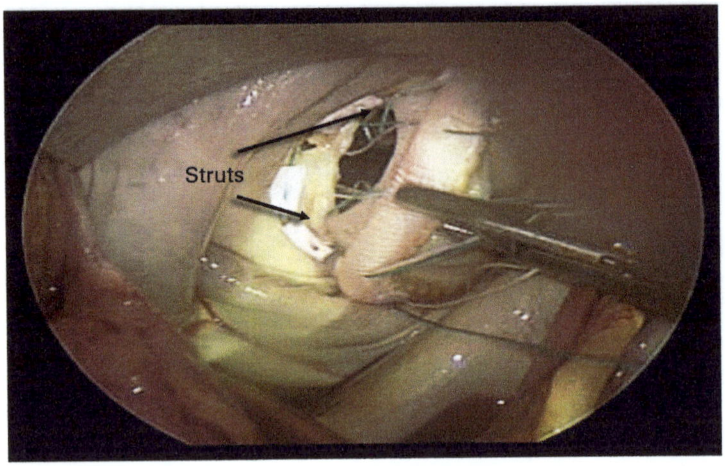

Fig. 5.53: After positioning the valve the correct placement of the struts has to be checked.

The implantation of a mechanical prosthesis seems to be simpler than a biological prosthesis. The reason is the necessity to check the position of the struts of a biological prosthesis. For that the holding mechanism should be removed at first. Now with two forcepses or a forceps and a hook the correct position of the struts can be seen (▶Fig. 5.53). Tying the knots should be started at the struts to fix the prosthesis in a correct position.

Using biological prostheses means the struts must be checked very careful before starting to tie the knots. With the videoscope an exact assessment of the situation is possible.

6 Tips and tricks

6.1 Perfusion's challenge

Depending on the type of perfusion, the management of flow, ventilation, and pressure plays an important role in avoiding cerebral injuries.

The standard procedure of retrograde perfusion starts before the thoracic cavity is opened. But what happens if ventilation is stopped at this time? There is a retrograde flow over the femoral artery with a defined level. But, of course, an antegrade flow still exists as long as the heart is not completely empty. This antegrade blood is not oxygenated anymore when ventilation is stopped. In the end, a zone with mixed retrograde oxygenated and antegrade nonoxygenated blood results (▶Fig. 6.1).

It is difficult to control how much oxygenated blood is in that zone and actually where the zone is located in the aorta. But for cerebral oxygenation it makes a dramatic difference if that zone is located in the ascending or descending aorta. The first situation leads to a normal oxygenation of the brain but the second may result in heavy damage.

All of this may be avoided by using the Estech EasyFlow direct aortic cannula, which will give antegrade flow. This alternative procedure was described exactly in Section 4.1.

The consequences are clear. While the heart is not completely unloaded and the perfusion is performed in a retrograde way, the ventilation should not be completely stopped. Only when a complete unloading of the heart is reached (and the pulse curve is flat on the screen) may ventilation be stopped. To check this moment effectively, a pressure line should be placed in the right radial artery.

To avoid these problems, ventilation should be performed side separated. With the use of a double lumen endotracheal tube the ventilation of the left lung may be continued as long as the heart is not completely unloaded (for details see Section 2.1).

The same problem may be found after declamping the aorta. When the heart starts to beat and is filled with blood, antegrade perfusion is started. Especially in order to verify the result of mitral valve repair, a transesophageal echocardiographic examination under physiological working conditions of the heart should be performed. This situation always leads to a significant antegrade flow of nonoxygenated blood if the lungs are still not ventilated. If this situation takes a few minutes, the oxygen saturation of the blood will decrease to critical levels with a high risk of cerebral damage.

The only way to avoid this critical situation is to ventilate the left lung while the antegrade blood flow is higher than the retrograde flow.

> If the decision was made to use retrograde arterial perfusion, a side-separated intubation and ventilation should be used. The ventilation of the left lung is needed at both the beginning and end of the operation.

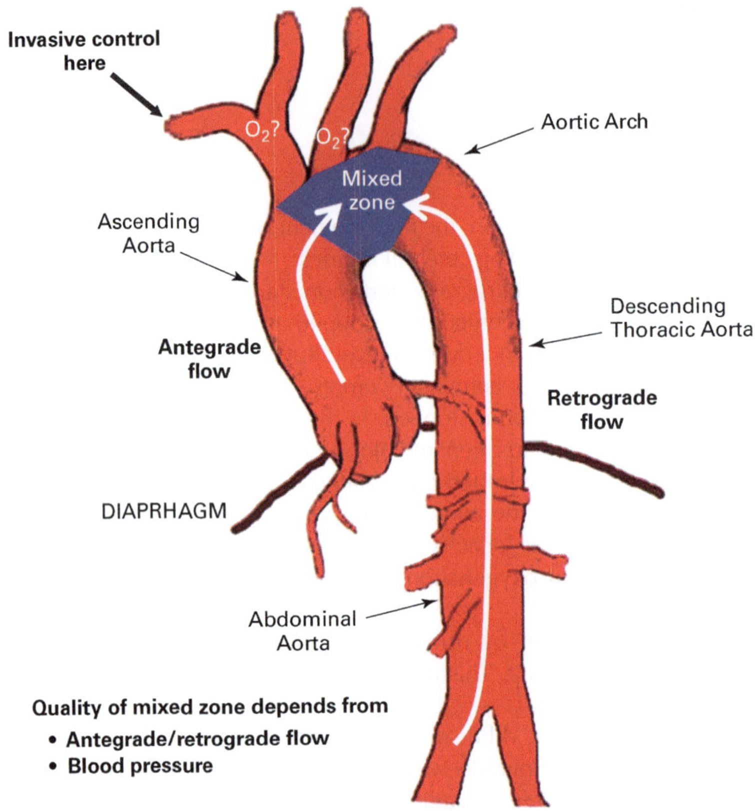

Fig. 6.1: The mixed zone results from a nonoxygenated antegrade flow and the retrograde flow over the arterial cannula.

6.2 Diaphragm's obesity

A diaphragm can never be too obese. But in two special situations the right diaphragm may block the way to the left atrium because of a huge bulge of the diaphragm that reaches the middle of the thoracic cavity.

The first situation is seen in patients with real obesity. If they lay on their back the intra-abdominal pressure will shift the diaphragm much higher than normal (▶Fig. 6.2). This can be expected. But sometimes the height of the diaphragm is surprising because it does not follow the body's constitution. Here, some anatomical particularities or a larger liver may play a role.

In both cases a heavy restriction for a direct view or for the way to the left atrium results. A safe way to get a better situation is to use a suture to pull back the diaphragm. The result is an open angle between the pericardium and the diaphragm with more space for the instruments and better control of the atriotomy. By the way, it prevents injury to the diaphragm through the knot pusher or other instruments.

To perform this suture, the first stitch goes through the muscle part of the diaphragm at the highest point of the bulge. It is absolutely important to imagine that the diaphragm is not thicker than 4 or 5 mm, sometimes less. This means that the stitches have

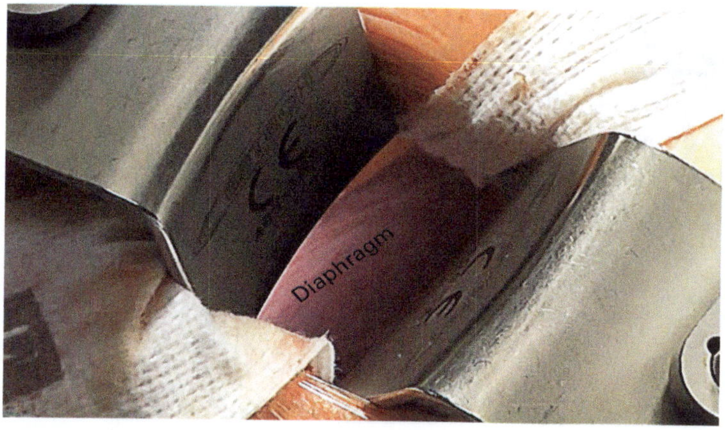

Fig. 6.2: Sometimes the diaphragm is seen in the middle of the thoracic cavity. In these cases the way to the mitral valve has to be cleared.

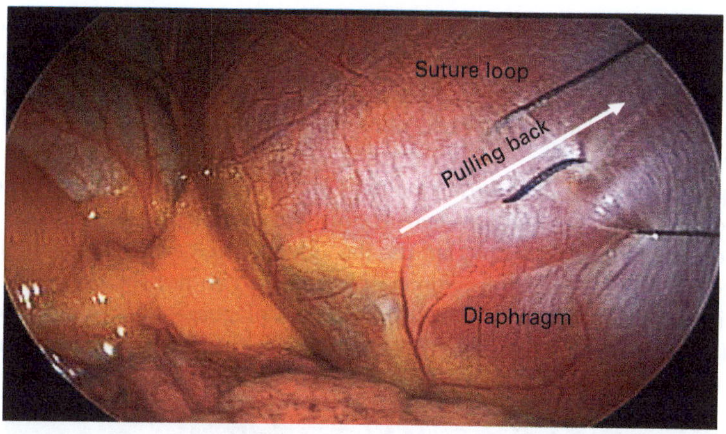

Fig. 6.3: For pulling back, a suture should be placed at the top of the diaphragm.

to be made very carefully, not deeper than 2 mm (▶Fig. 6.3). To get enough material for the tension, this stitch should be performed doubly. Then the suture may go through the skin or may be tied around a branch of the retractor. With increasing tension the diaphragm will be pulled back until the thoracic wall is reached (▶Fig. 6.4).

In some cases the diaphragm blocks the way to the valve. With a simple suture through the highest point that will be used for pulling back the diaphragm, the situation becomes more comfortable.

6.3 View's hurdles

Regardless of the size of the thoracic incision and the anatomical situation, some reasons exist for getting a bad view to the aorta, the left atrium, or the mitral valve.

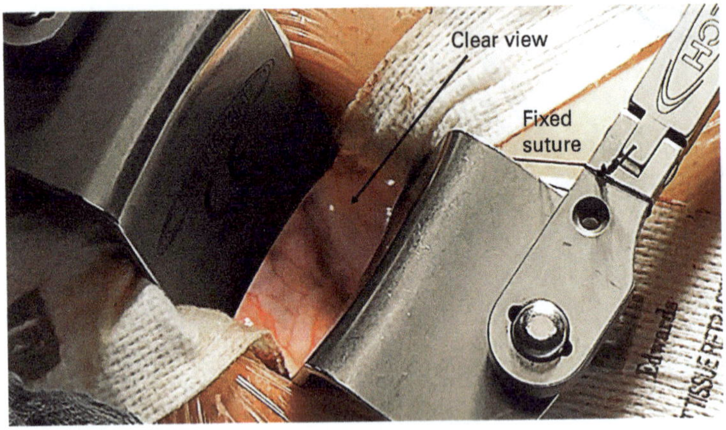

Fig. 6.4: After pulling back until the lateral thoracic wall is reached a clear view to the heart and the mitral valve is possible.

Some special descriptions for placement of the videoscopic camera, the position of the diaphragm, and the incision at the thoracic wall were made in corresponding chapters (see Chapter 4, Sections 4.2 and 4.4). Nevertheless, in some cases all compliance with recommendations and tricks does not seem to help get a comfortable view to the structures inside.

At this point, let's face it, it doesn't matter. Do not try to search for the "perfect view" for one hour only to find out that there is no such thing. If you can not see the aorta directly because it seems to be too far, use the videoscopic camera and/or try to change the intercostal space used. If the videoscopic camera can not show you the incisions from the inner side, pull it back from their original placement and move it trough the thoracic incision by hand (▶Fig. 6.5). If there is a fold inside the left atrium and it is

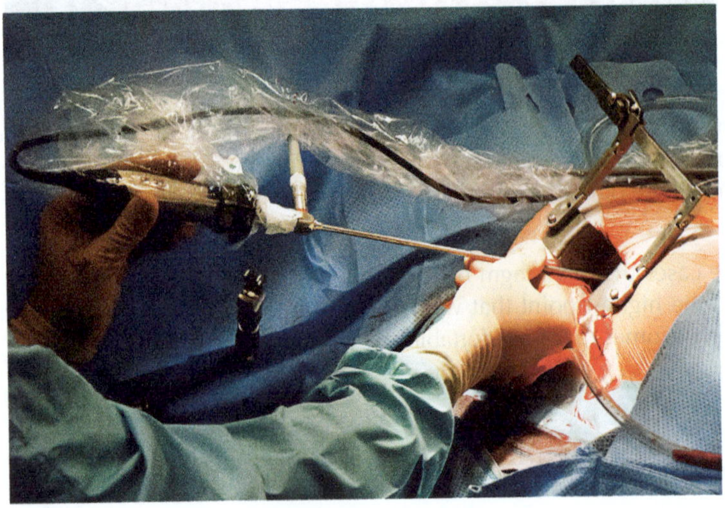

Fig. 6.5: Change the scope position and use by hand to check the stitch incisions from the inner side of the thoracic wall.

impossible to see the posterior part of the annulus clearly, make the atrial incision a bit larger and the fold will be smaller.

The mystery to reaching a comfortable situation in every patient is not to install a standard situation at every price but, rather, to install a standard situation with flexibility. This is similar to many other situations in cardiac surgery. If one wants to make a coronary bypass grafting it is clear before the operation which coronary artery should be grafted. But during surgery one has to choose very accurately which segment is the right or the best one.

Like all parts of an endoscopic procedure, getting an acceptable view depends on many details. Take enough time to clear the camera if necessary. Change the direction of the 30°optical system as long as needed to see what you want.

At the end, the best way to overcome the hurdles for a nice view is to combine the direct with a monitor picture. With some of the described tricks, one can expect in every patient an optical access to carry out the operation under controlled and safe conditions. Surprisingly, in most patients the working conditions become more and more favorable despite the primary conditions if the operation goes on.

Using an endoscopic technique for mitral valve repair lives depends on an excellent view despite a small thoracic incision. Some small additional steps can help get a nearly perfect situation. But sometimes this cannot be reached – do not spend too much time improving a nonimprovable situation.

6.4 Instruments' versatility

All surgical instruments have a special field of use. Additionally, hand-dependent use is often found (i.e. everybody knows the bad function of a scissors in the left hand). Because of this, in open heart surgery a "multiple functional use" of instruments is not common. If one needs another instrument the scrub nurse will give it and if one needs another hand an assistant will lend one. This is completely different from an endoscopic situation.

Here, a small number of special instruments is available, and the main construction type is always the same (see Section 3.3). Except for some fixed supporting technical structures (i.e. the atrial hook) there is an opportunity for the simultaneous use of two instruments only without any additional help. Because of these limitations some special technical features are helpful.

One of the important features is the use of the knot pusher. It is important enough for the quality of results and the performance of the operation to devote a special chapter to this instrument (see Section 6.5).

With all other instruments every opportunity should be taken to use them in more than one functional field. The typical situations for this are the closure of a leaflet after resection of a prolapse, the implantation of Neochord, and the implantation of artificial rings (for technical details see Chapter 5). In all of these cases, a situation will be reached that is characterized through tissue holding with a forceps in the left hand and starting a stitch with a needle of a suture to perform the nextstep (▶Fig. 6.6). Regardless of the concrete technical situation, in an endoscopic approach under these conditions the forceps has to be used to pull out the needle. However, if it does so, the forceps has to let go off the tissue because there is no other means of support and the result will be a completely changed and reduced view and a bad orientation.

This unfavorable situation may lead to a time-consuming attempt to get the result of a procedural step or to a compromise in quality. To avoid this, the functional capacity of the instruments has to be extended with additional ideas for use.

What does this mean? Primarily, the surgeon's view on endoscopic instruments has to enlarge. Do not see in a needle holder a needle holder only. With the same instrument and the stitched needle in the tissue, the system of needle holder and needle may achieve a forceps-like or assistant-like function. It is simple to lift up the tip of the papillary muscle with the needle holder if the needle is stitched in (▶Fig. 6.7).

The same holds true for artificial ring sutures, especially behind a tissue fold in the region between 3:00 and 7:00 (▶Fig. 6.8). Here, the first step may be a stitch with the

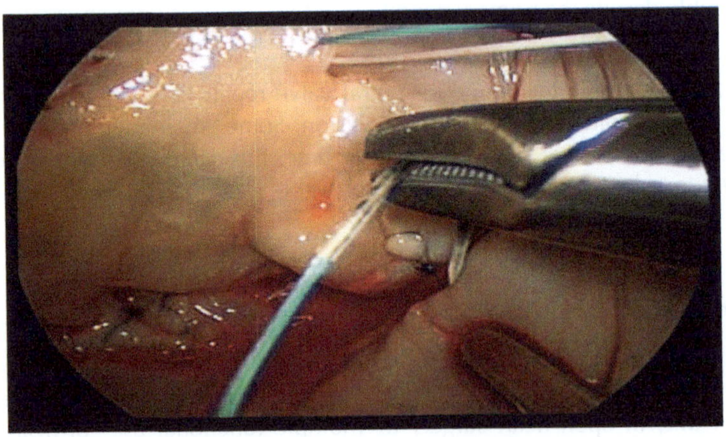

Fig. 6.6: To start the suturing of tissue the forceps keeps the tissue and the needle holder makes the first stitch. No other help is available.

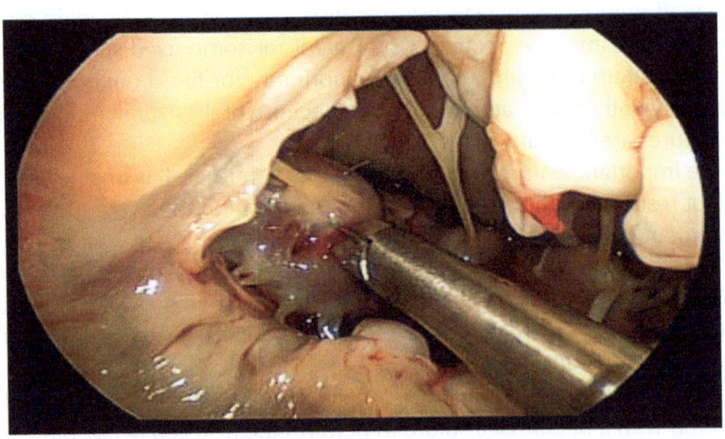

Fig. 6.7: Using a stitched needle for an "assistant-like" function.

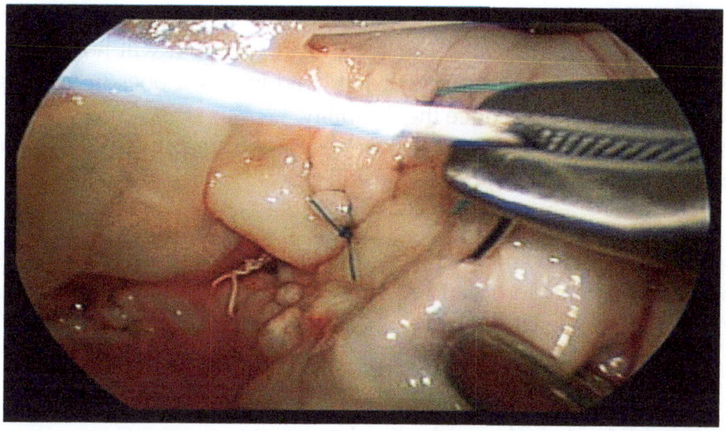

Fig. 6.8: For placement of sutures near the posterior ring it might be advantageous to use the needle at first to pull back the tissue a bit. Then the tissue may be fixed with the forceps and the stitch may be placed exactly.

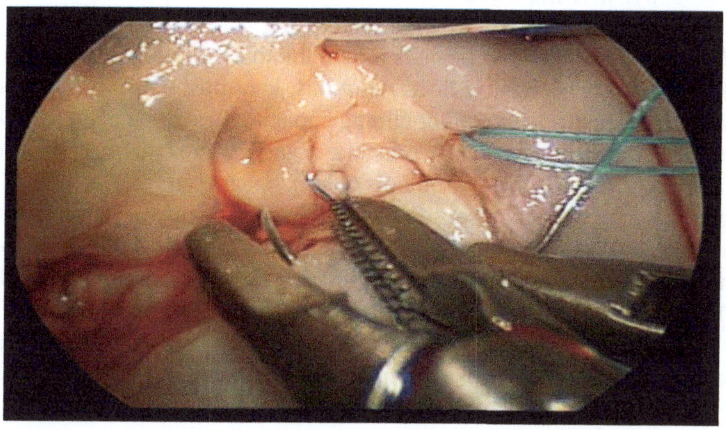

Fig. 6.9: Typical change of function between needle holder and forceps. After performing the stitch the forceps can let off the tissue and may be used to keep the needle out.

needle into the tissue near the planned final suture placement to pull back this region a bit with the system of needle and needle holder. Then, with the forceps in the left hand, the atrial tissue may be fixed at this point. Using this procedure the fold is now out of the direction of the view and at least under a clear view (direct or videoscopic) the needle may be stitched in the right position. Then follows the same step as described previously – the needle holder lifts up the tissue and the forceps may be used to pull out the needle, letting off the previously fixed tissue (▶Fig. 6.9).

Another difference is the nonhand-dependent use of instruments. In some cases it is necessary to work more on the left side of the valve, for example, on segment A1 or P1 or in the vicinity of them. Here, often the classic situation with the forceps in the left hand and the scissors in the right is uncomfortable because the instruments have to cross each other to work or they block the view. This situation is easily solved with a change of the instruments from hand to hand. A "reverse classic instrument handling" results, but in contrast to instruments in open heart surgery it will not affect the functional quality. The scissors works in your left hand just as it does in your right – it is your training only that might reduce the flexibility.

Under this mental attitude, with every new case the surgeon's skills in endoscopic surgery and the flexibility to reach the goal will grow.

> The instruments that are made for endoscopic surgery seem to have the same function as instruments for open heart surgery. But additional functions can be learned for comfortable working.

6.5 The knot pusher's independent existence

An absolute must for endoscopic mitral valve surgery is the knot pusher. This instrument allows a knot to be tied in the depth of the thoracic cavity that cannot be reached manually. It is the basis for every step in endoscopic mitral valve surgery (▶Fig. 6.10).

Some different models of knot pushers are on the market, but for practical use a safe and simple handling is necessary. Because of this, knot pushers with a simple mechanism to catch the suture and excellent gliding capacities are advantageous. One of the best seems to be a mechanism that works like a gliding loop that can be opened and closed as a forceps (e.g. see the instruments of Estech, San Ramon, CA, USA).

Although the working mechanism seems to be simple, the quality of the knots and routine use of the knot pusher include some technical tricks. Despite using the knot pusher as recommended, the results could be not satisfied. It seems as if there is an "independent character" of the knot pusher despite the formally correct use by the surgeon.

Everybody knows how a suture has to be tied into a knot in open heart surgery. And if one imagines the movements of both hands while a knot is tied it will be very clear what the function of a knot pusher in endoscopic surgery is.

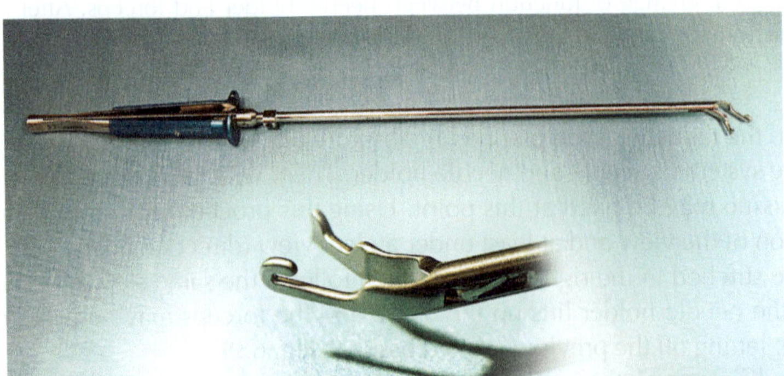

Fig. 6.10: An example for a model of a knot pusher. The detailed picture of the tip shows the mechanism for catching the suture. With a simple one-hand-working mechanism the eye may be opened and closed (Estech, San Ramon, CA, USA, 2009).

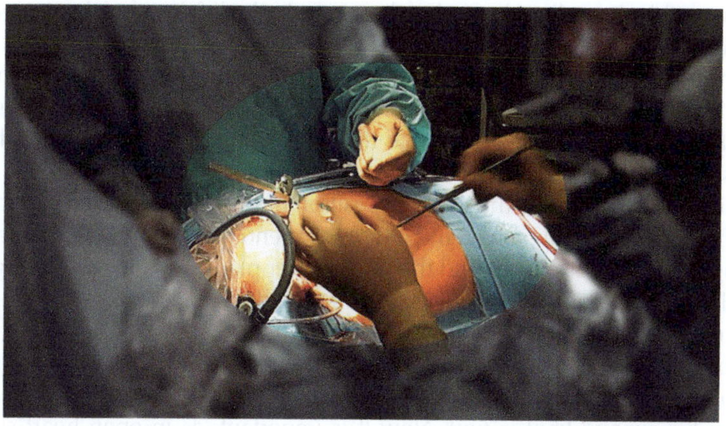

Fig. 6.11: The left hand of the surgeon holds the left end of the suture while the right hand uses the knot pusher. An assistant keeps the right end of the suture under low tension.

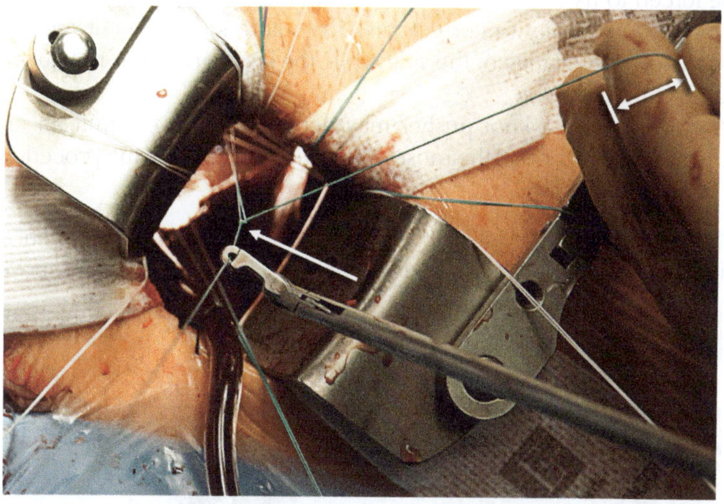

Fig. 6.12: While the surgeon moves the knot pusher inside the thorax the assistant keeps his or her end of the suture somewhat tight.

Because of the fact that use of the knot pusher means that the left hand keeps one end of the suture and the right hand moves the knot pusher, another hand is necessary to keep the other end of the suture (▶Fig. 6.11).

Then the forward movement of the knot pusher imitates the right hand of the surgeon to push the knot down into the thoracic cavity.

For the first moment it seems as if the hand of the assistant has to bring his or her end of the suture under tension so the knot can glide down. This is not true. That is not its function. The assistant has only to keep his or her end of the suture somewhat tight so that the knot is able to glide. If the tension is too high the knot will not glide, especially in twisted sutures such as those for ring implantation and also in Prolene® or Cardionyl® sutures (▶Fig. 6.12).

Opposite to this, in reality, the end of the suture in the left hand of the surgeon has to be under increasing tension while the knot is being pushed down so the knot will stay in the right position at the end. While moving the knot pusher down, the instrument has to be brought into an position opposite to the end of the suture that the surgeon's left hand holds (and takes the suture that the hand of the assistant holds with itself to cross the surgeon's end) (▶Fig. 6.13).

Why this move? It leads at the definite position of the knot to a situation to pull the knot tightly. At the end of this movement the suture end in the surgeon's left hand is positioned right to the knot pusher and the knot pusher plays the role of one finger of the right hand of the surgeon in open heart surgery to tighten the knot. The assistant should (and can) never do this (▶Fig. 6.14).

This procedure has to be repeated for every knot and should be exercised as often as it takes to become a routine. The main meaning of this special movement becomes clear when the second knot is tied. Now it is important (as in open heart surgery) to tighten both knots, but this will not succeed when the knot pusher is at the false side. This does not matter for the first knot, but in this situation with the second knot the first one will be forced to fix above the desired position (so-called air knots). In most cases there will be no opportunity to correct this. The suture has to be cut out and another one has to replace it. A change of the side while the knots are tied is not necessary if six knots are used at minimum.

In the end, the use of a knot pusher may accelerate or even limit an endoscopic operation. It seems to be one of the most underestimated parts of the procedure.

A knot pusher is a very special instrument. Because an additional (assistant's) hand is needed to tie a knot, it works correctly with a complex pattern of movements only.

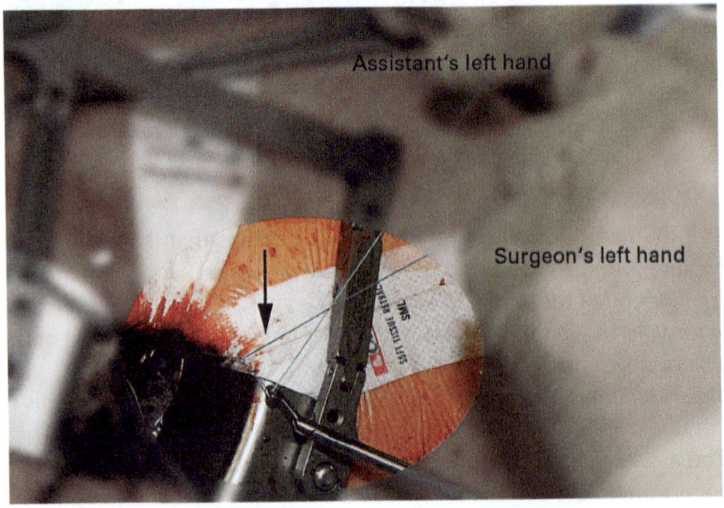

Fig. 6.13: On its way, the knot pusher has to cross the left end (surgeon's end) of the suture and take the right end with itself.

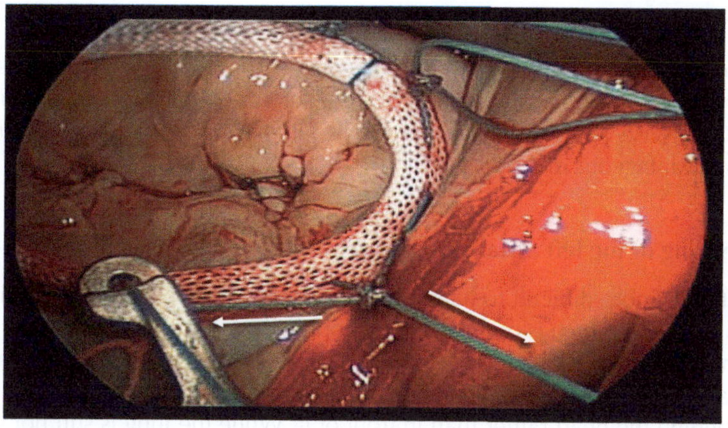

Fig. 6.14: After crossing the left end of the suture the knot pusher will be the "one finger of the right hand" of the surgeon inside the thorax and should tighten the knot while the left hand of the surgeon keeps the left end of the suture under tension.

6.6 Managing bleeding

One of the main characteristics of endoscopic surgery is the low traumatizing effect of the procedure. The small thoracic incisions and the only two active injuries of anatomical structures (the needle in the ascending aorta and the incision in the left atrium) cause, in general, a low risk of bleeding.

Nevertheless, there are some additional opportunities for bleeding. All of them result primarily from injuries to the surrounding tissue at different times and for different reasons. Mainly, these are a bleeding out of the left atrial appendage, an injury to the right pulmonary main stem, an injury to the right mammary artery, and a bleeding from intercostal arteries.

6.6.1 Bleeding of ascending aorta

For the cardioplegic system, the aspiration of the aorta is necessary. To control this situation after removing the needle a pledget-supported suture is prepared. Sometimes the aortic wall is thin or calcified and a closure of the aspiration hole does not succeed with the prepared suture. This is not so dangerous. To control the situation and to stop the bleeding an additional suture with pledgets may be used (i.e. Prolene 3 x 0 or 4 x 0 with an SH1-needle).

For relieving the aorta and a safe closure it is better to relieve the heart and to decrease the blood pressure. If that is not enough, the heart should fibrillate again and the aorta may be cross-clamped for a short time. If the situation is not clear to demonstrate hemostasis, do not hesitate to remove all sutures and start again. Sometimes the circumferential hematoma or fatty tissue may make the situation confusing. In these cases it is better to remove all sutures and start again than to try to stop the bleeding with wrongly placed sutures again and again.

6.6.2 Bleeding of the left atrial incision

This normally is the simplest situation for bleeding. If there is a bleeding of vessels from the atrial tissue (caused by preparation of the interatrial septum), coagulation may be enough. Otherwise an additional suture will help. Bringing the suture in retrieving volume is advantageous in most cases.

6.6.3 Bleeding of the left atrial appendage

This situation is more difficult to handle with endoscopic access. The reason is a localization of bleeding, which is opposite to the approach.

Bleeding out of the left atrial appendage will be seen at the end of the procedure. After restarting the heart and circulation, an ongoing quantity of blood will be seen, which is behind the heart rather than in front of it. While the lung is still not ventilated this blood is typically dark. After restarting the ventilation it becomes bright red.

The reason for this bleeding is in most cases a hole that is caused by the aortic clamp. If the clamp is not rotated with the curved tip toward the head, this tip may catch the thin wall of left atrial appendage. One will never feel it, but there is bleeding at the end. So the rotation of the clamp may avoid this complication very reliably (for details see Section 4.6). Another reason might be a manipulation of the left atrial appendage from inside the atrium. Closing the appendage can lead to a defect that will not be seen as long as the atrium is open.

To solve the problem in most cases, the conversion to sternotomy and to suturing the hole is the best way. It is safer, simple, and time-saving. Another way is to fibrillate the heart again, to reopen the left atrium and to try suturing the defect from the inside. But for control of the result all steps have to be performed again and if there is still a bleeding …

6.6.4 Injury of the right pulmonary main stem

This is another embarrassing complication that will be caused by too deep a stitch at the left angle of atrial incision. The needle reaches the pulmonary artery, the suture will be tied into a knot, and a small injury of the right pulmonary main stem results. The appearance of the bleeding is the same as if it comes out of the left atrial appendage, but the origin may be not found. Sometimes it seems to be a bleeding out of the left atrium and one will be tempted to reopen it and close it again. Typically the bleeding will reappear and every additional stitch will worsen the situation.

In the end, a conversion to sternotomy and solving the problem from the anterior is the only way for success in most cases.

> The injury of the right pulmonary main stem is difficult to handle through endoscopic access. To solve the problem a conversion to sternotomy is indicated.

It should be clear that the injury of the pulmonary artery is avoided very simply. It is enough to think of it when suturing the atrial incision's left angle is carried out. Sometimes it may be necessary to prepare the space between the atrial wall and surrounding tissue a bit. It is not necessary to demonstrate the right pulmonary main stem. It shows again that in contrast to open heart surgery the way back has to be carried out as carefully as the way to the valve.

6.6.5 Injury of the right mammary artery

The most common reason for a bleeding out of the right mammary artery is the use of the atrial hook. The stick to keep the blade in position goes through the thoracic wall, and if the necessary incision is too close to the sternum (i.e. to the middle of the thorax) bleeding starts from the injured artery. Sometimes there is a small bleeding only (i.e. a side branch) but it goes on and on after the end of surgery and may cause a re-thoracotomy.

Because the exact position of the mammary artery is mostly unknown, there is always a certain risk of injuring this vessel. Therefore, it is absolutely necessary to check this area before the small thoracotomy will be closed.

> A bleeding out of the right mammary artery is mostly caused by the atrial hook only. Therefore, this area has to be controlled absolutely before the small thoracic incision is closed.

The best way to do this is through a videoscopic inspection. Because of the mobility of the camera and the flexible direction of view through a 30° optical system, every area opposite to the lateral wall may be viewed and a bleeding may be demonstrated. The necessary measures against the bleeding are the same as in open heart surgery. They also can be carried out with the help of the videoscope.

6.6.6 Bleeding of the intercostal artery

This kind of bleeding is the most malicious. It starts often after removing the port for the optical system or the additional working port. One may not be able to inspect the inner side of the lateral thoracic wall directly or by means of the optical system. So after the end of surgery some blood will be collected in the thoracic cavity and a re-thoracotomy has to be performed. This is the reason to inspect the inner side of the lateral wall with the hand-held optical system as a matter of routine, which means to remove the camera from the stabilizer and bring it in through the mini-thoracotomy. Then it is easy to rotate and move the camera in every direction that is necessary to verify all points of the perforation of an intercostal space.

> Bleeding of an intercostal artery often only becomes apparent after all ports have been removed. To control these perforations of the thoracic wall the optical system should be removed from the stabilizer for manual use through the mini-thoracotomy.

For safety and to avoid later bleeding out of the tissue channels, a nice trick may be used. In every heart surgery unit the use of Tabotamp® is common. The package is normally rolled and may be cut in the middle. Then an absorbable suture may be used to

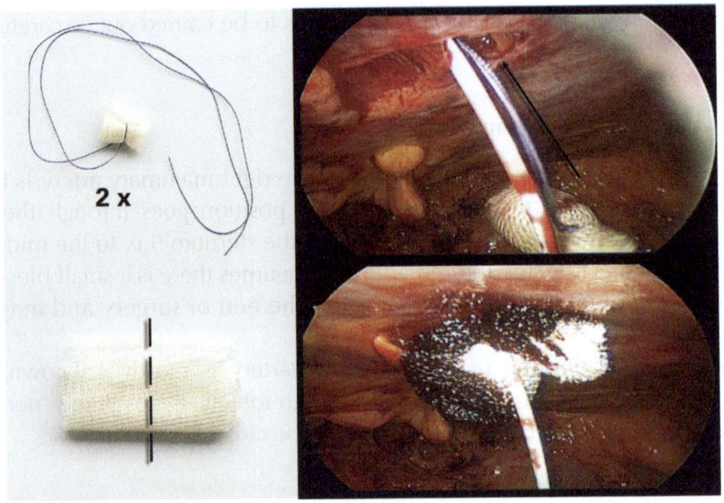

Fig. 6.15: A half package of Tabotamp® was fixed by an absorbable suture (left). After pulling back the ends through the small perforations the suture can be used for closure and to fix the Tabotamp® on the inside (here: closure of the hole made for the scope).

fix this half of a role as it is. With a small clamp the ends of the suture can be pulled back through the small incision to the outside, and the suture may be fixed subcutaneously. With this procedure the piece of Tabotamb® will close the perforation from the inside and a bleeding will be stopped or not develop (▶Fig. 6.15). It is recommended to use this small procedure for thoracic perforations made for the atrial hook and the port of the scope as a matter of routine.

7 Additional procedures

7.1 Left atrial ablation

Mitral valve insufficiency is often combined with atrial fibrillation. The reason may be the ongoing volume stress of the atrium with enlargement of the diameter, increased wall stress, and even structural wall changes that support a rotational excitation. For more details see the numerous articles in the literature.

Besides the well-known classic Maze procedure, interventional and surgical techniques were developed in the past few years to isolate the foci of these excitations. Other than by the physical energy used, the surgical methods may be divided into endocardial and epicardial procedures. For endoscopic surgery both methods may be used, but there are some differences in handling and result.

7.1.1 Endocardial ablation

This type of ablation is mainly characterized through the energy directed from the inside to the outside. It is clear that this ablation type can only be used in patients whose left atrium has been opened. Therefore, the combination of a mitral valve repair with an endocardial ablation seems to be logical. But for practical use, some disadvantages will become apparent concerning the type of physical energy that is used.

Using the unipolar radio frequency technique leads to the necessity to avoid esophageal injuries. One of the main preventive procedures is to bring isolating material such as a compress or a rubber glove behind the posterior wall of the left atrium. This is not a simple procedure for an endoscopic approach, but it is necessary to avoid incorrect energy directions.

The other problem is to achieve a perfect line around the pulmonary veins and to the mitral valve to get a complete lesion set. As a special feature of endoscopic mitral valve repair, and in contrast to open heart surgery, the bottom of the left atrium is not clearly visible; neither directly nor with the videoscopic technique. This means a noncontrolled way around the pulmonary veins if a pen-like or a longer flexible stick will be used. In both situations and regardless of the physical energy used tissue folds may cause gaps in the line (▶Fig. 7.1).

Another problem seems to be a higher rate of patients with an AV block after cryogenics. The reason may be a damage of the surrounding tissue, for example, the AV node. The use of cryogenics means to freeze the tissue with a temperature of –160°C for 120 seconds. The idea is a deep destruction of the atrial tissue where the probe is in the contact area. The direction from the inside to the outside may provoke the damage to the tissue behind the atrial wall. The effect of this technique and for this use is relatively uncontrolled and is based on the idea: "to finish off all with one big shot" (▶Fig. 7.2).

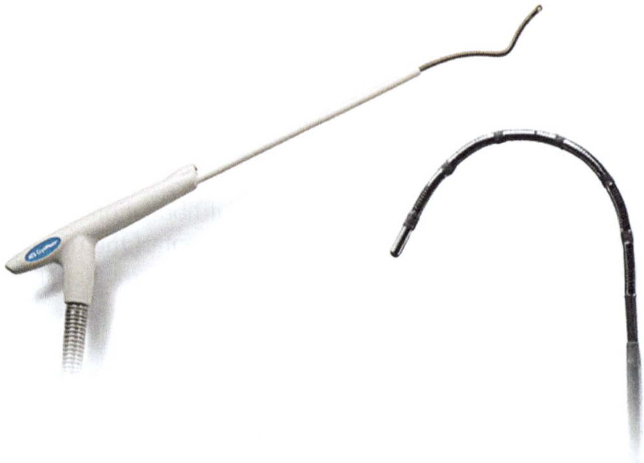

Fig. 7.1: Typical probes for endocardial ablation. As well as the probe for cryogenics (Cryocath; left) the probe for radio frequency (Estech, San Ramon, CA, USA, 2009; right) is flexible and may be adapted to the size and shape of the atrium.

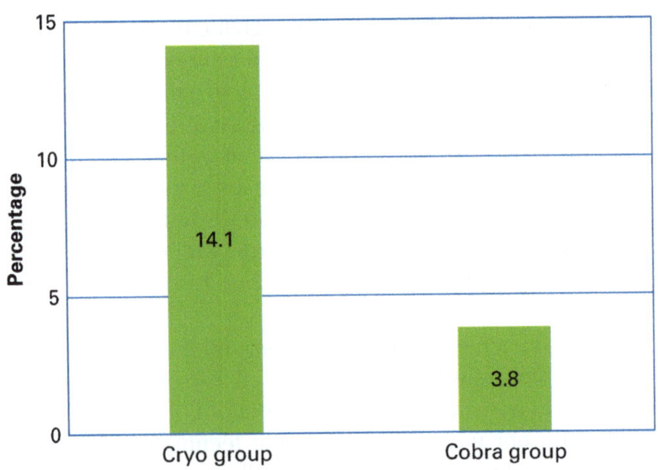

Fig. 7.2: Need for pacemaker implantation after endocardial ablation. A significantly higher number after using cryogenics were seen (in percent, cryo-group n = 78; RF group n = 48, author's own results).

Endoscopic endocardial ablation is often combined with an uncontrolled way around the pulmonary veins. For cryo-technique, a higher rate of pacemaker implantations was seen.

The practical advantage of endocardial ablation is the opportunity to do more than a box lesion alone. There is an ongoing discussion about the necessity of additional lines

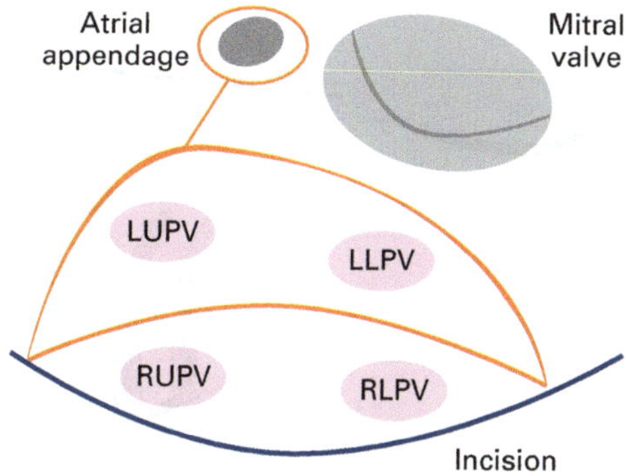

Fig. 7.3: Typical pattern of lines for endocardial ablation. The line to the mitral valve and the typical line between the pulmonary veins should improve the results.

to reach the best results or to improve the overall results. It has not been resolved whether the mitral line is necessary and it is still less clear whether an additional line around the orifice of the left atrial appendage is necessary. To follow all these ideas a complex pattern of lines was developed for endocardial ablation (▶Fig. 7.3).

For practical use, longer and flexible devices have been preferred over the past few years. They allow working on longer distances with a shorter time for the overall procedure. For best results it seems to be important to avoid tissue folds with gaps in the end. For this the wall may be tensed a bit with a forceps and the device should be brought into stable contact with the endocardial tissue layer.

For the use of cryogenics, a simple trick helps avoid tissue damage posterior to the left atrium. If cooling of the device was started some frozen adhesions between the device and the tissue will be seen. Now the device may be lifted up a bit and so the posterior wall of the atrium will follow this movement, and contact between the frozen tissue and the structures behind the posterior wall may be avoided.

The advantage of an endocardial ablation is to make more than a box lesion alone. Nevertheless, the risk of gaps is higher if an endoscopic technique is used.

7.1.2 Epicardial ablation – pulmonary veins clamp technique

The technology of clamping the pulmonary veins does not matter in connection with the endoscopic mitral valve surgery. Because of the completeness and because this procedure is very important in open heart surgery, here the basic principles should be imaged (▶Fig. 7.4).

The main idea of this technique is the isolated ablation of right and left pulmonary vein orifices after preparation and clamping with a special ablation tool. Theoretical background is the well-known study of Hassaguere, which showed that the origin of ectopic additional stimulating processes may be found at the transition between pulmonary veins and the left atrium.

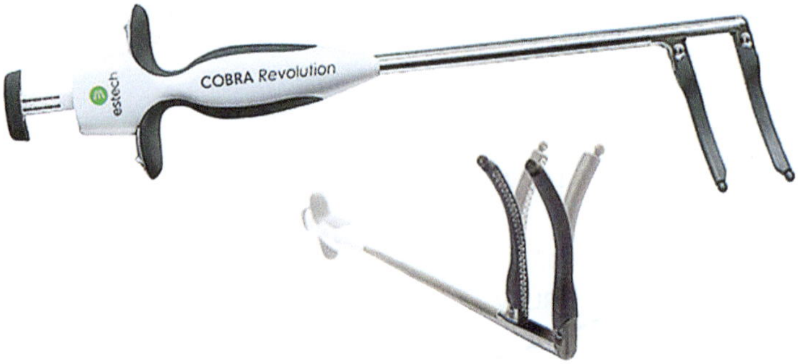

Fig. 7.4: Typical example of an epicardial ablation clamp (Estech, San Ramon, CA, USA). The easily rotatable branches allow a simple switch from the left to the right side and back.

In practical performance the pulmonary veins will not be clamped but the parts of the left atrial wall that are attached to the pulmonary veins directly.

Besides, the inclusion of the atrial wall in the ablation area seems to have two advantages: On the one hand, the area isolated by the ablation is bigger than with an isolated ablation of the veins themselves. On the other hand, the risk of developing pulmonary vein stenosis as a result of the ablation becomes significantly lower.

The epicardial technique of ablation using clamps is recommended for open heart surgery only. For one-side endoscopic access, this procedure is not recommended.

For all other details of this procedure, see the special literature and the product description.

7.1.3 Epicardial ablation – box lesion with Cobra Adhere XL®

Today the epicardial unipolar atrial ablation by means of radiofrequency is one of the standard procedures for simultaneous ablation during endoscopic mitral valve procedures. The basic principle is to create a box lesion that completely encloses the connections between pulmonary veins and the left atrium. Because adding other lines is realizable only with bigger expenses, the discussion originated over and over again during the past years with regard to the question of whether the box lesion alone is enough. Results of my own comparative studies show that by careful execution of the procedure, a high success rate is to be registered (▶Fig. 7.5). On this occasion, the successful reconstruction of the mitral valve may play a supporting role.

Over the past years, a growing number of cardiac surgeons and electrophysiologists have learned to work together on chronic atrial fibrillation. The main idea is to use a combined therapeutic strategy consisting of a surgical epicardial ablation as a box lesion and interventional added lines in the left and/or right atrium. The advantages are an overall time-saving combined procedure and a potential improvement of the results

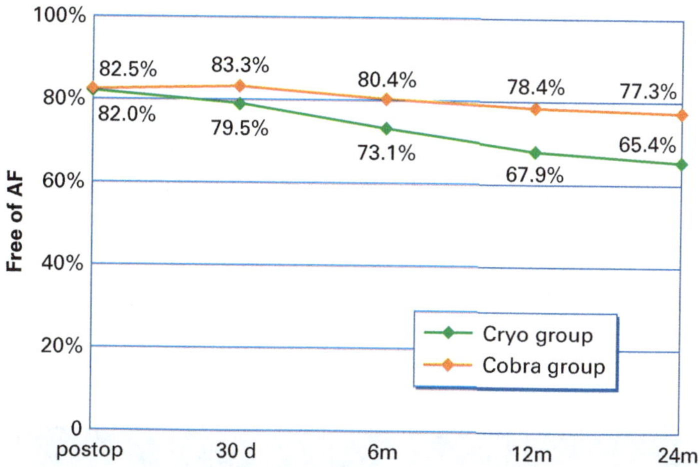

Fig. 7.5: Twenty-four-month time course of the results after epicardial ablation (Cobra Adhere XL) and endocardial cryo-ablation. The results show a small decrease of the rate of patients without atrial fibrillation and a larger decrease in the cryo-group (author's own results).

with a more successful therapy for patients with chronic atrial fibrillation. A basic condition is the endoscopic endocardial ablation.

An essential condition for the successful application of a tool for an endoscopic epicardial ablation is the easy and safe introduction of the ablation device. Presently the tool Cobra Adhere XL® from the company Estech (Estech, San Ramon, CA, USA) is the only device that fulfils these requirements. Because the understanding of the technical background for the successful application is essential, a quick introduction follows.

The epicardial ablation with a flexible tool that can be used from the right side alone is the technique of choice for endoscopic ablation today. The tool Cobra Adhere XL® is currently the only one on the market.

Technical background of Cobra Adhere XL®

One of the main qualities of the device is its distinctive flexibility. It is the condition for the very easy and safe guidance of the tool around the pulmonary veins. After the correct placement the probe will be fixed on the outside of the atrial wall by means of suction. A stable and effective contact between the electrodes of the probe and the tissue surface results at the same time. The continuous cooling with a salt solution during the procedure allows the application of high amounts of energy without the risk of damaging the surrounding tissue. The essential qualities are shown in ▶Table 7.1.

The device applies the energy at about radio frequency. Using a total of 10 electrodes the energy is applied in groups to a maximum of 5 electrodes. The duration and the temperature to be reached are freely eligible so that a sure transmurality can be reached. For further details, see the product description and information of the company Estech.

Table 7.1: Main characteristics of the device Cobra Adhere XL® (Estech, San Ramon, CA, USA).

Characteristics	Description
Flexibility	Enables easy and safe placement and free handling of the tool
Suction	Holds Cobra XL in the right position around the pulmonary veins and preserves an excellent contact between tissue and tool
Cooling	Temperature in the deep of the tissue is above 60°C – surface cooling prevents additional damage
Effectiveness	Radio frequency in combination with suction, cooling, and temperature control allows a reliable transmurality (overcomes heat sink effect)

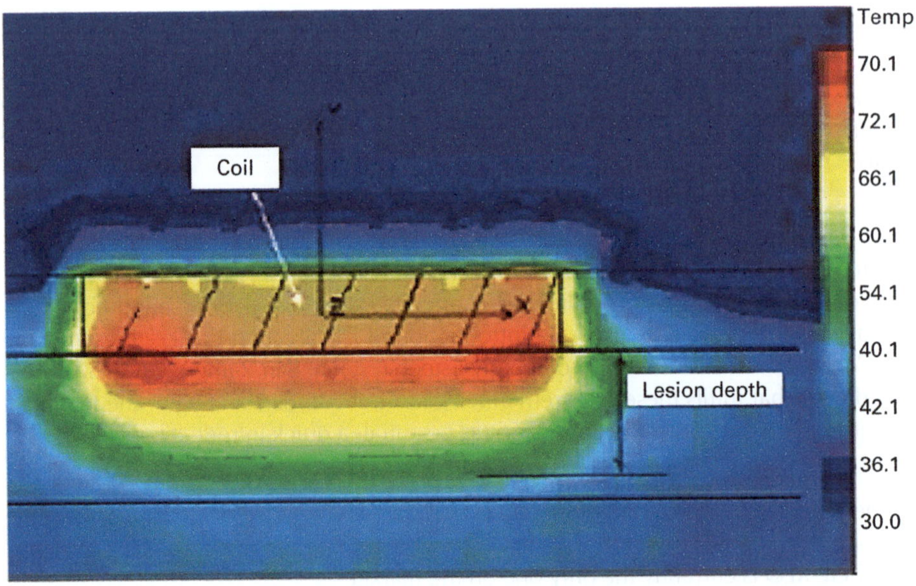

Fig. 7.6: The applied energy leads to a temperature of more than 50°C inside the tissue. The closer you get to the inner layer the more the temperature sinks (heat sink effect). To overcome this effect, more energy has to be applied (with permission from Estech).

Heat sink effect

The impairment of the temperature inside the atrial tissue from epicardial to endocardial in epicardial ablation procedures is named the heat sink effect (▶Fig. 7.6). The goal of energy application is to reach a temperature of more than 50°C in the complete thickness of the wall. The blood inside will act as cooling fluid and so a layer of lower temperatures will be found near the endocardium. To overcome this heat sink effect (and to achieve transmurality), applying more energy is necessary. To avoid damage to the surrounding tissue, the cooling of the surface is helpful (▶Fig. 7.7). This is one of the main advantages of using a tool like Cobra Adhere XL®.

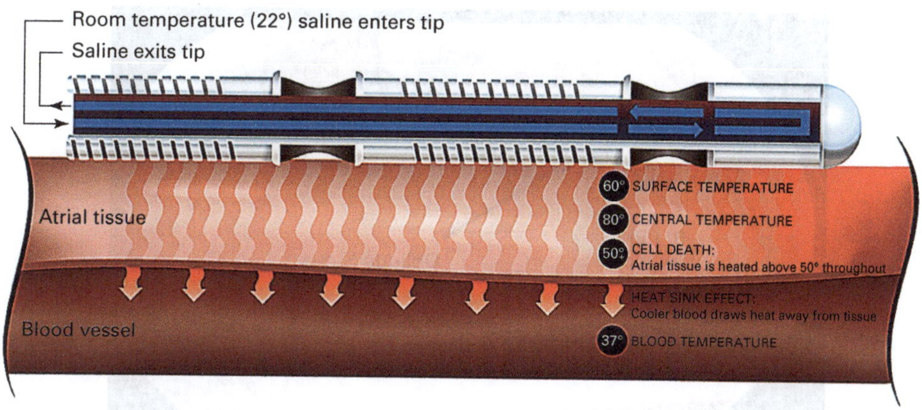

Fig. 7.7: The principle of cooling for applying more energy. Cooling at the outside of the atrial wall allows transporting more energy into the tissue to overcome the heat sink effect (with permission from Estech).

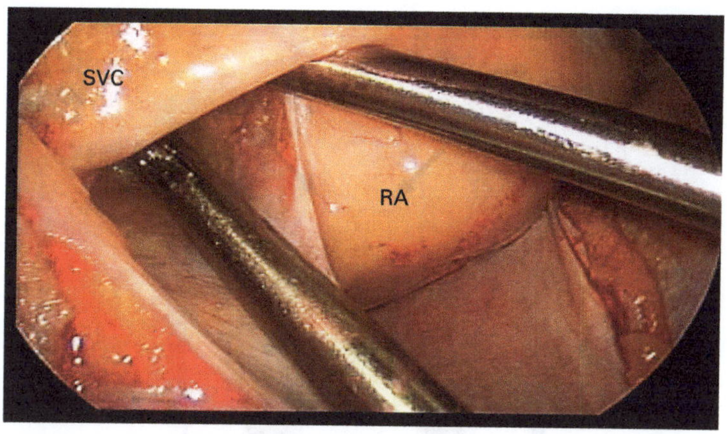

Fig. 7.8: A typical endoscopic situation to prepare the way between superior vena cava (SVC) and right upper (RA) pulmonary vein.

Practical use of Cobra Adhere XL®

For endoscopic use of Cobra Adhere XL® an introducer system is necessary. A newer two-tailed system includes two flexible guiding poles with magnetic tips. After preparation of the oblique sinus and transversal sinus, the stretched poles can be introduced (▶Fig. 7.8, ▶Fig. 7.9, ▶Fig. 7.10).

After pulling back the guidewires the flexible parts meet and the magnetic tips will be connected (▶Fig. 7.11). A complete loop around the pulmonary veins is the result.

> The basic of using Cobra Adhere XL is the preparation of the natural way around the pulmonary veins. An introducer system simplifies the application of the tool.

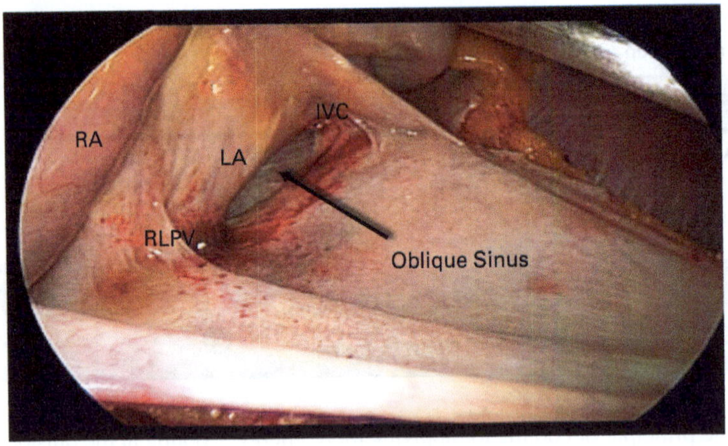

Fig. 7.9: The preparation between inferior vena cava (IVC) and right lower pulmonary vein (RLPV) is normally simple but has to be carried out very carefully. Bleeding out of the posterior wall of the vena cava must be avoided.

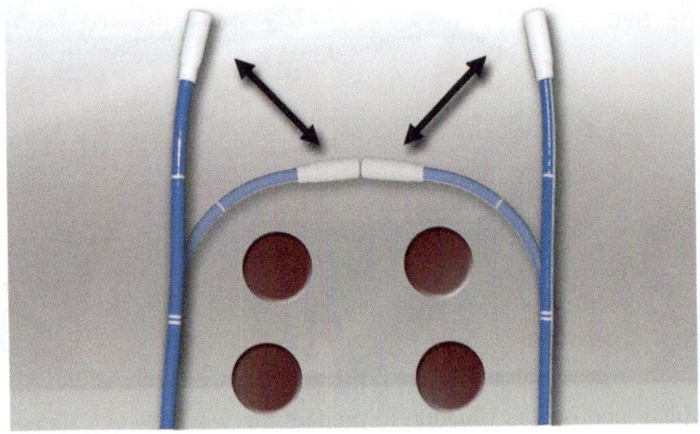

Fig. 7.10: The two-tailed introducer system contains the guiding tools with magnetic tips. After inserting the guidewires the tools will be stretched.

After connecting it with one end of the introducers and pulling it through the complete introducer system the probe can be placed around the pulmonary veins. With the TEE the correct positioning of the probe (above the left atrial appendage) has to be checked. Then the suction can be started and the probe stably placed (▶Fig. 7.12). Ablation can be started with defined parameters.

A good filling of the heart is necessary for a sufficient and stable contact between the surface of the left atrial wall and the probe. Therefore, in patients with already started extracorporeal circulation, the heart should be refilled. But remember: The procedure described here is a beating-heart procedure regardless of extracorporeal circulation has been started. Do not use the epicardial monopolar radio frequency ablation in empty hearts or after applying cardioplegia.

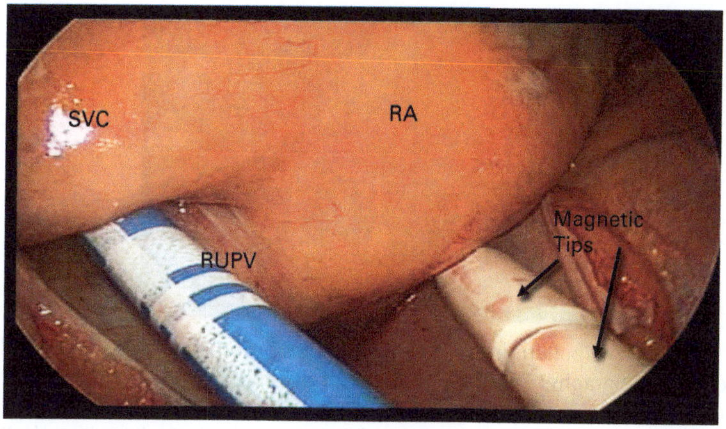

Fig. 7.11: After pulling back the guidewires the tools will create a loop behind the left pulmonary veins. The magnetic tips meet and connect the tools. (RA: right atrium; SVC: superior vena cava; RUPV: right upper pulmonary vein)

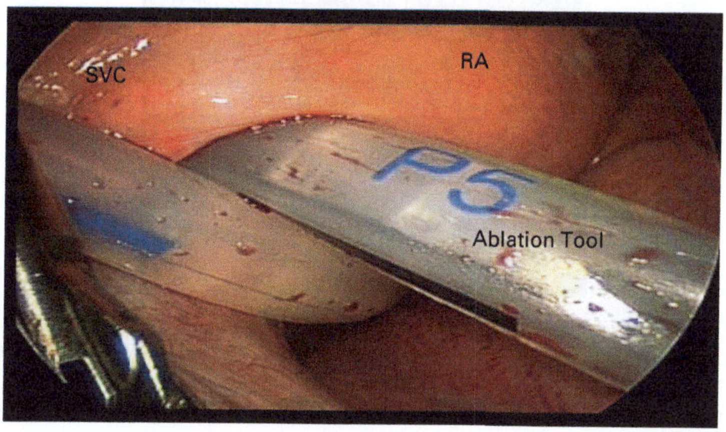

Fig. 7.12: The loop of the tool around the pulmonary veins is finished. After checking the correct position, suction can be started to fix the tool on the epicardial surface. Then the ablation can be started. (RA: right atrium; SVC: superior vena cava)

> Checking the position of the tool by TEE before starting with the ablation and the use in filled beating hearts only are the main conditions for a very safe and reliable function.

7.2 Management of the left atrial appendage

Mitral valve insufficiency is often combined with atrial fibrillation and needs atrial ablation. In these cases the necessity to close the left atrial appendage will be discussed.

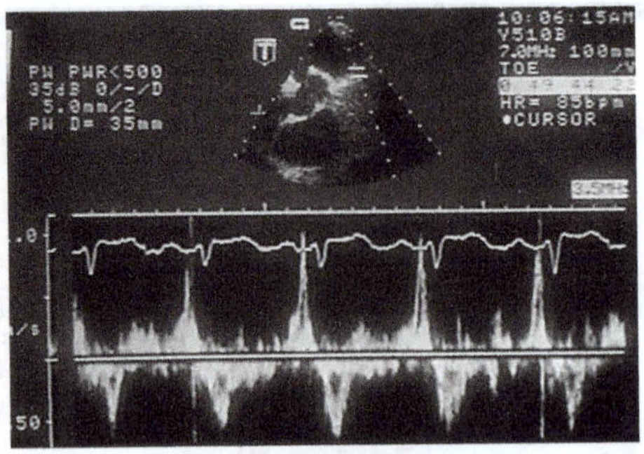

Fig. 7.13: Typical flow pattern in a left atrial appendage in patients with a sinus rhythm detected by echocardiography. The clear phase of inflow and outflow is the main factor in finding no thrombus inside the appendage (with permission from N. M. Al-Saady, O. A. Obel, A. J. Camm: Left atrial appendage: structure, function, and role in thromboembolism, *Heart* 1999;82:547–555).

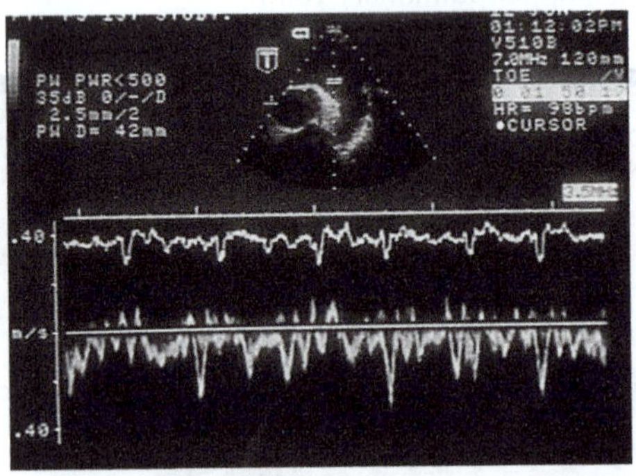

Fig. 7.14: In cases of atrial fibrillation the flow pattern is completely changed. No clear inflow and outflow will be found. The risk of developing thrombi is very high (with permission from N. M. Al-Saady, O. A. Obel, A. J. Camm: Left atrial appendage: structure, function, and role in thromboembolism, *Heart* 1999;82:547–555).

A flow pattern that includes both an inflow and an outflow phase can be seen in the left atrial appendage in patients with a sinus rhythm by echocardiography (▶Fig. 7.13). In cases with atrial fibrillation this flow pattern is changed to an irregular and nonphasic flow without a clear movement of the blood inside the appendage (▶Fig. 7.14).

Results of different studies have shown a benefit for prevention of a neurological stroke when the appendage was closed. But today it seems to be clear that this beneficial effect depends on the shape of the orifice of the appendage. At the end the discussion follows the question about whether there is enough blood flow to get a wash-out effect.

The existence of a wash-out effect in patients with atrial fibrillation corresponds to the diameter and the shape of the orifice. The larger the orifice and the shorter the appendage itself the more the effect of the blood flow leading to a lower risk of a thrombogenic formation. In contrast to this finding, a smaller and longer appendage shows normally no or little blood flow only with a high possibility of thrombus development. Former studies have shown that the diameter of the orifice is age dependent (▶Fig. 7.15).

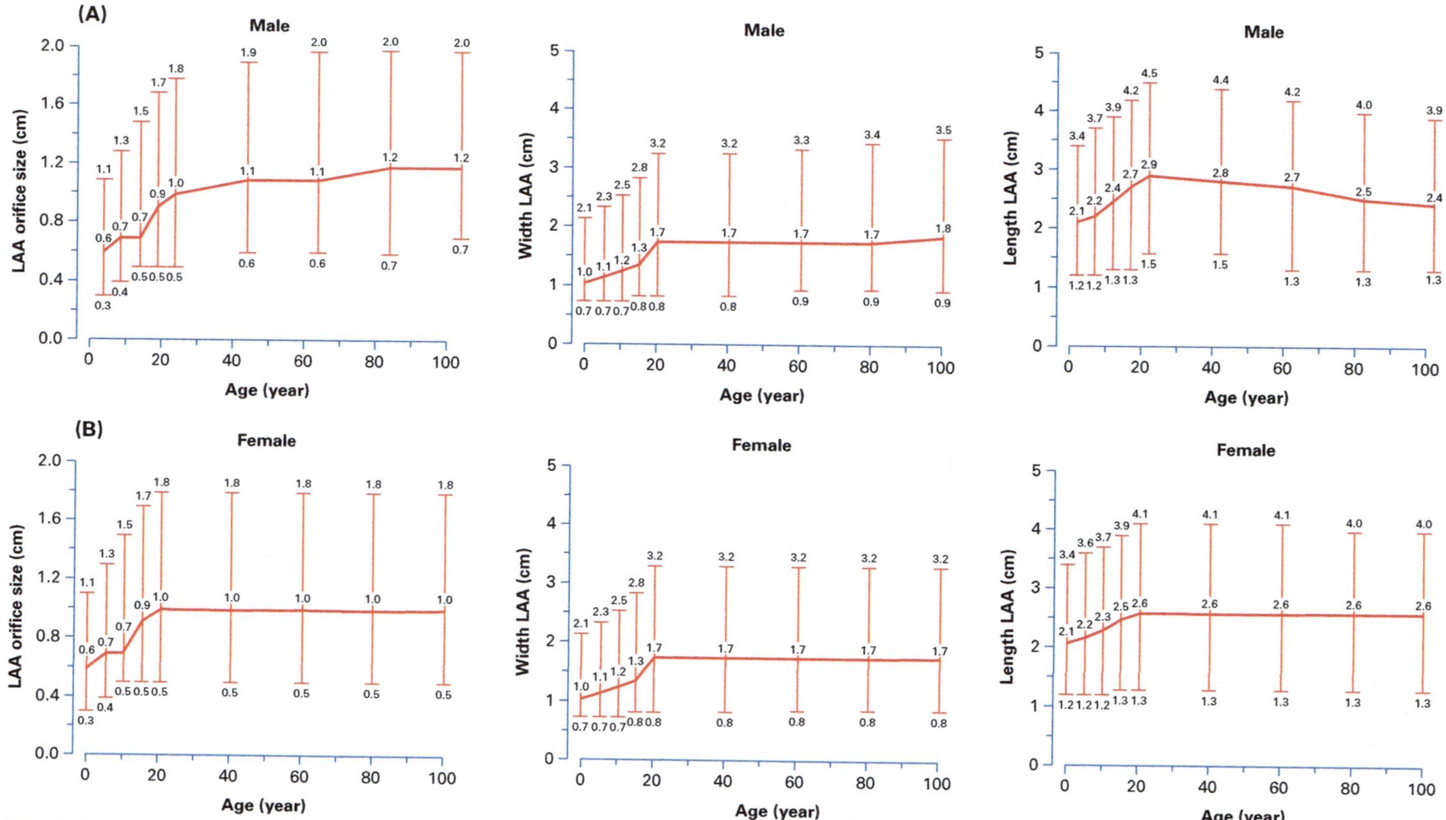

Fig. 7.15: Parameters as the diameter of the orifice as well as width and length describe the anatomical characteristic feature of the left atrial appendage. The change of these parameters with age seems to be more relevant in males (with permission from Veinot, J. P. et al. *Circulation* 1997;96:3112–3115).

Depending on these conditions it seems to be clear that the closure of an atrial appendage should be recommended in every case with a small orifice. There is no measure regarding when the orifice is small enough for necessary closure, but the shape will be identified more comfortably with growing experience.

The closure of the left atrial appendage seems to be necessary in appendages with a small orifice and a longer length. The individual anatomical situation seems to change with age.

In cases of an unclear situation, the decision should lead to a closure of the appendage. At the end it is the only possibility to prevent a thromboembolic event.

As a helpful tool for decision making, the $CHADS_2$-score was developed. This score allows estimating the risk of developing a thromboembolic event in patients with atrial fibrillation (see ▶Tables 7.2 and 7.3).

For practical reasons, it should be advantageous to close the orifice of the appendage before the repair starts because of the normally used artificial ring, which may interfere with a safe closure of the appendage.

For closure, a 3 x 0 Prolene suture can be used. A smaller needle is better than a larger one. A durable closure is the condition for a lasting prevention of thrombi. So at first, a circular suture that goes around the orifice will tighten the orifice very well.

Table 7.2: The $CHADS_2$-score weights risk factors for developing a stroke.

Risk factor	Description	Points
C	Congestive heart failure	1
H	Hypertension	1
A	Age	1
D	Diabetes	1
S2	Former stroke	2

Table 7.3: With an increasing number of points that result from the $CHADS_2$-score, the risk of suffering from a stroke within a year grows.

Points	Stroke risk (%)	95% – Confidential interval
0	1.9	1.2–3.0
1	2.8	2.0–3.8
2	4.0	3.1–5.1
3	5.9	4.6–7.3
4	8.5	6.3–11.1
5	12.5	8.2–17.5
6	18.2	10.5–27.4

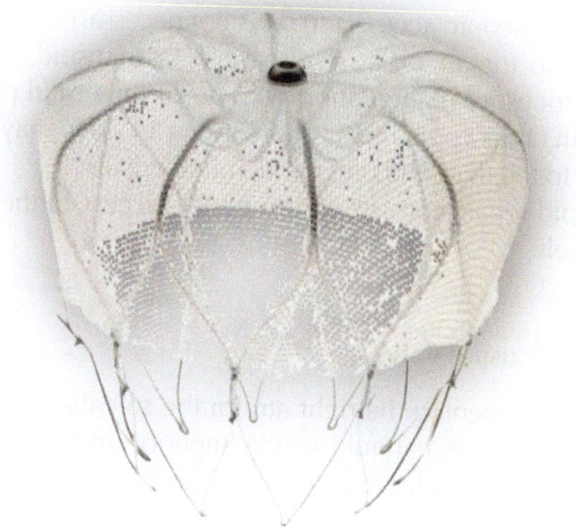

Fig. 7.16: Mechanical system for closing the left atrial appendage (example: Watchman®; Atritech Inc.; Plymouth, MN, U.S.A.).

Because of tissue folds another running suture should be used for an additional closure. The tissue has to be handled very carefully because it is sometimes very thin and bleeding out of the base of the appendage after declamping of the aorta could be seen. A reopening of the left atrium to stop the bleeding or a conversion to sternotomy would be the result (see also Section 6.6).

> The $CHADS_2$-score allows an estimation of the risk to suffer from stroke in patients with atrial fibrillation. If the decision for closure on the appendage was made, the closure should be carried out before mitral valve repair. It must be done very carefully (to avoid any bleeding at the end).

Newer developments show the possibility of closing the appendage using mechanical systems from the inside and clips from the outside. This technology allows closing the appendage with a stable mechanical system (▶Fig. 7.16). However, because of a lack of long-term data, a general recommendation to use this system cannot be given at this time. It is still unclear whether the antithrombotic effect corresponds to the one known from a closure by suture.

7.3 Tricuspid valve repair

In about 10% of all patients with mitral valve regurgitation, a tricuspid regurgitation also develops. The number seems to decrease because of a shorter time between diagnosis of mitral valve disease and operative repair of it.

Nevertheless, in cases with a higher graded tricuspid regurgitation, a repair of the tricuspid valve should be carried out. This procedure is simple to do and is very efficient in preventing an additional operation for tricuspid regurgitation later on. For discussion of operative strategy it should be clear that an additional repair of a tricuspid valve can be realized with an endoscopic access and does not necessarily need a sternotomy.

The same holds true for an isolated disease of a tricuspid valve. Some patients develop an isolated tricuspid regurgitation with no or only mild pulmonary hypertension. In these cases an endoscopic repair of the tricuspid valve may be very helpful and can prevent damage to the liver and other abdominal organs.

Endoscopic tricuspid repair consists of two parts – access to the tricuspid valve and repair of the valve itself.

7.3.1 Access to the tricuspid valve

It is well known that for opening the right atrium the so-called total bypass is needed. This means to have a venous cannula in the superior and inferior vena cava while turning off the right atrium. Similar to open heart surgery it is normally achieved with a ligature around the vena cava cannulas near the confluence to the right atrium.

But there are some differences. The first is the use of a cannula that is going through the right atrium to the superior vena cava. It is an advantage using a single cannula for the drainage of venous blood out of both the inferior and superior vena cava (for details of the cannula see Section 4.1).

For snaring the vena cava around the cannula it is necessary to prepare the way around the cavae similar to open heart surgery. Around the superior vena cava near the right atrium the hemiazygos vein (at the posterior part) and the nearby anatomical structure of the left pulmonary artery must be respected. With careful use of the scissors, the adhesions between the superior vena cava and the structures around may be cut and then with a long curved instrument, such as a clamp after Overholt, a band for snaring may be brought around (▶Fig. 7.17).

The same procedure is applicable for snaring the inferior vena cava. Here an instrument with a larger curve should be used. For preventing complex bleeding out of the posterior part of the inferior vena cava the preparation should be carried out very carefully.

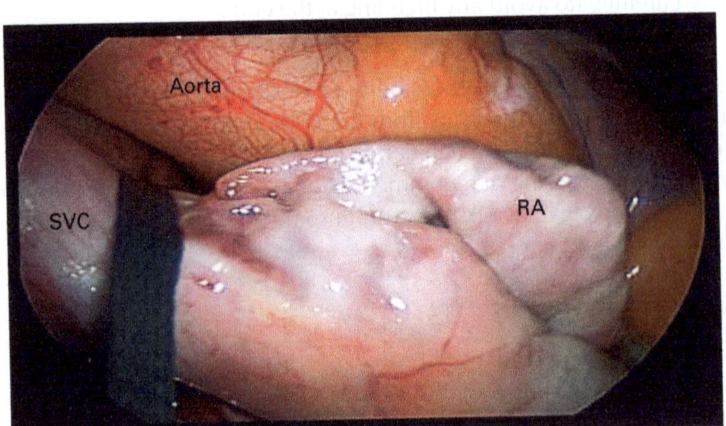

Fig. 7.17: A band for snaring is brought around the superior vena cava. (RA: right atrium; SVC: superior vena cava)

In contrast to open heart surgery the snaring itself will be performed a bit differently. If one uses a clamp to keep the snaring band in the right position, this clamp would stay in the way to the right atrium or the tricuspid valve. To avoid this situation a clamp should not be used. With a little trick it is possible to bring in the snaring bands into the thoracic cavity without interfering with the instruments.

For accessing the valve, a snaring of both venae cavae is needed. A venous cannula with two inlet areas allows simple handling.

To perform the snaring the sleeve for the band has to be shortened to a length of about 5 cm. Then a small wadding can be brought between the two ends of the band and the band can be tied over the wadding (▶Fig. 7.18). Then the two ends may be

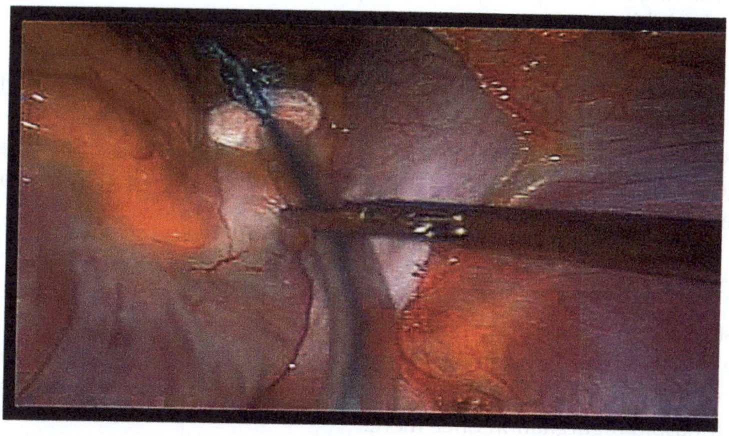

Fig. 7.18: To snare the vena cava the band was tied over a small wadding. Then the complete snare may be brought into the thoracic cavity.

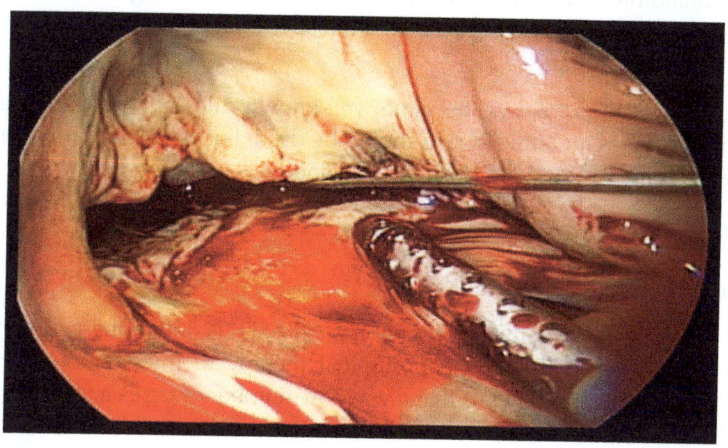

Fig. 7.19: The atrial hook keeps the roof of the right atrium. With the scope, the presentation of the tricuspid valve is relatively simple.

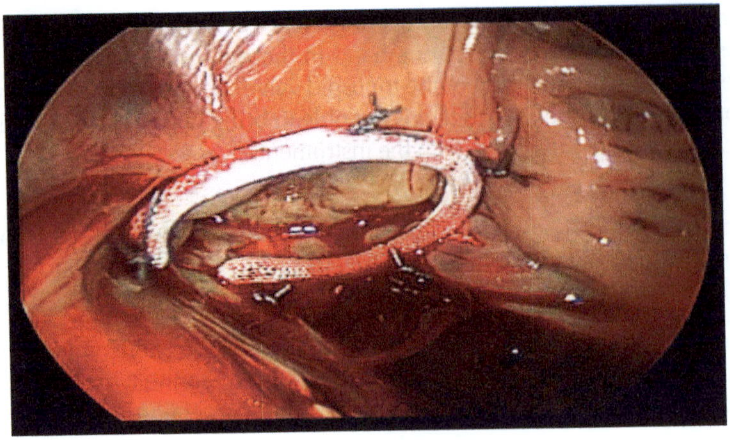

Fig. 7.20: The ring for tricuspid repair was implanted. The gap to avoid damage to the AV node is clearly visible.

shortened and the complete snare may be lowered into the thoracic cavity. If the two snares are handled as described, the way to the tricuspid valve is free.

The next step is the opening of the right atrium. The incision is the same as in open heart surgery. In order to inspect the valve the smallest atrial hook (see Section 3.3) or two sutures may be used. It is relatively simple to get a good view (▶Fig. 7.19).

7.3.2 Repair technique

In contrast to mitral valve repair the tricuspid repair focuses more on the narrowing of the native ring. For that the well-known De-Vega-plastic or similar techniques may be used. Recent results have shown that the use of an artificial ring is advantageous to prevent a tricuspid regurgitation once more.

The ring implantation follows the same rules as in open heart surgery for positioning and as for artificial ring implantation in mitral valve surgery, which was described. Mainly the anatomical relation between the native tricuspid ring and the AV node is important to avoid an AV block at the end of the operation (▶Fig. 7.20).

The repair technique follows the same well-known rules as for open heart surgery. In most cases an artificial ring should be used. For closure of the atrial wall an inverting suture may avoid multiple bleeding.

7.4 Closure of the ASD

The atrial septal defect type II (here simply named ASD) is one of the issues in the past few years that has shifted from heart surgical therapy to interventional procedures made by cardiologists. This means that a very low number of cases a year for necessary surgical closure of an ASD are presented.

However, if it is necessary to close an ASD using an operation, the sternotomy of the mostly younger patients should be avoided. For these otherwise mostly completely healthy patients, the scar of a complete sternotomy is a stigma for life. An endoscopic approach should be the access of choice because of its atraumatic nature.

7.4.1 Technical considerations

Coming from the right thoracic side an ASD is more problematic to see than from above. Therefore, the thoracic access should be more anterior. The intercostal space that will be used is the same as for endoscopic mitral valve surgery (see Section 4.2).

It is clear that for opening the right atrium, a snaring of both vena cava is necessary as described in Section 7.3.

The necessity of preparations for the use of cardioplegia depends on the situation of the patient and the preferences of the surgeon. Normally cardioplegia is not necessary and the procedure is performed under cardiac fibrillation. If cardioplegia should be used the preparation, follow the rules described in Section 4.5.

7.4.2 Closure of the ASD

After opening the right atrium with an incision at typical localization one or two sutures may be used for keeping the atrial wall out of view. A flexible sucker should be brought into the orifice of the sinus venosus (▶Fig. 7.21).

With an additional thread that is going around the cannula (remember: the flexible cannula goes through the right atrium into the superior vena cava), the cannula itself can be pulled a bit to the side. This is sometimes necessary when the ASD is a bit larger or the localization is more lateral (▶Fig. 7.22). In these cases the cannula may partially block the view to the ASD.

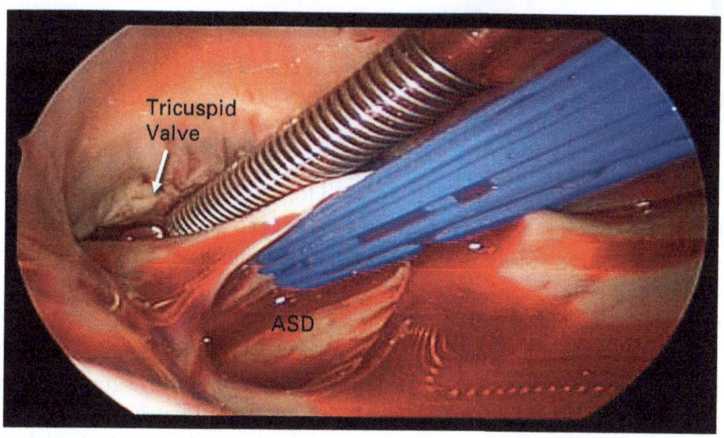

Fig. 7.21: Typical setup for endoscopic closure of an ASD. A suture pulls back the atrial wall and a flexible sucker is positioned in the orifice of the sinus venosus. The ASD is found relatively central to the sinus.

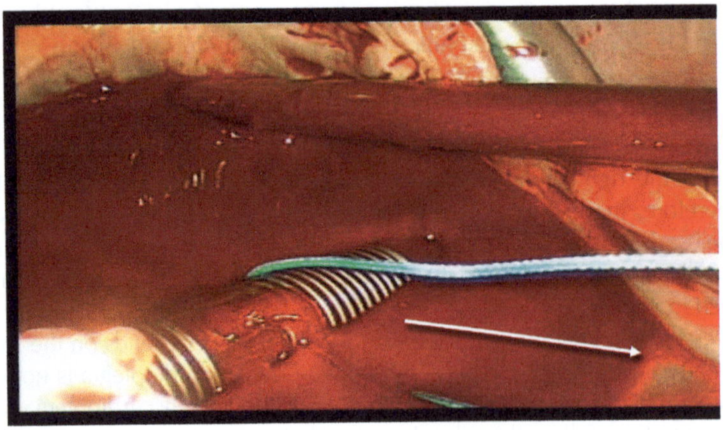

Fig. 7.22: A thread pulls the cannula to the side. The view of the ASD is not blocked.

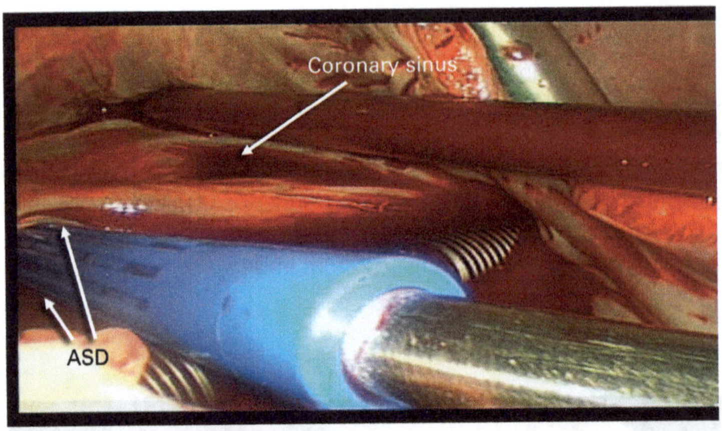

Fig. 7.23: The atrial septal defect type II is normally found relatively central. Sometimes the orifice of the sinus venosus is found nearby (arrows).

It does not matter which technique is applied for closure. Both the direct closure and the implantation of a patch is possible using endoscopic access.

Closure with a running suture alone is simple. In order to obtain the optimal result it is necessary to identify the ASD exactly. It means not to fail with the partial or total closure of sinus venosus, which may sometimes be found very close to the ASD (▶Fig. 7.23).

For a larger ASD, the closure using a pericardial patch is the common technique. In cases with a pulmonary vein that brings the blood to the right atrium the patch has to be used for canalizing the blood to the left side. Normally it is known before the operation starts but in some cases a surprising situation will be found.

After identifying the anatomy the patch can be properly sized. It seems to be advantageous to fix the patch with two sutures at the poles. With every end, a running suture to the middle part of the patch should be performed (▶Fig. 7.24).

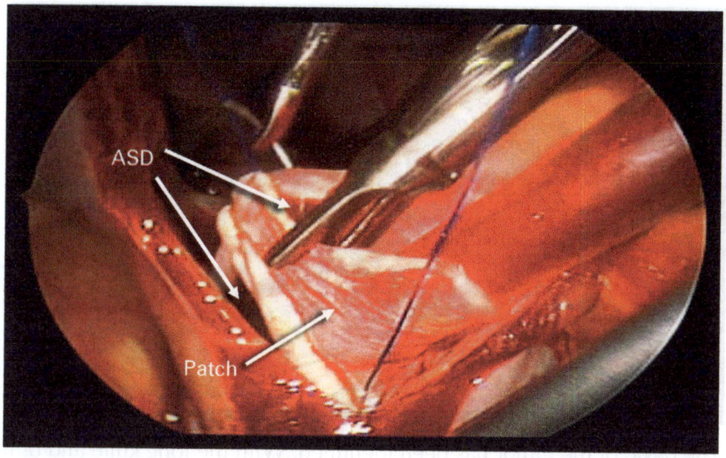

Fig. 7.24: Closure of an ASD with a patch. Running sutures from every pole make it simple to bring the patch in to the right position.

The access follows the same rules as described for tricuspid repair. The direct closure of an ASD is very simple. For implantation of a patch the limits of the ASD should be defined very exactly.

7.5 Excision of left atrial tumors

The tumors inside the left atrium are in most cases myxomas. Typically these tumors have a stem and a larger and movable head. The size differs from cherry-like to very large orange-sized tumors. Therefore, the removal of the tumor can be achieved by cutting out the stem under a clear view or by removing a tumor that fills out the left atrial cavity. The tumor may occasionally even partially fall out once the atrial wall is opened.

In most cases the stem is localized near the septum but in very few instances all areas might include a tumor stem. In rare cases the tumor is localized not in the atrium but in the left ventricle. Normally it is not a problem to work through the mitral valve in the left ventricle and it seems to be simpler than after using a classic sternotomy.

7.5.1 Theoretical remarks

The stem of a myxoma grows out of the endocardial tissue. For preventing the tumor from growing back later it is necessary to cut it out with a part of the endocardial tissue. This may sometimes lead to a wall or septum defect. But normally it is very simple to close the defects with a direct suture.

Tumors localized inside the left ventricle especially may have a histology that is different to a myxoma. In these cases an intraoperative first histological examination of the cut-out tissue may help to make a decision for a larger excision.

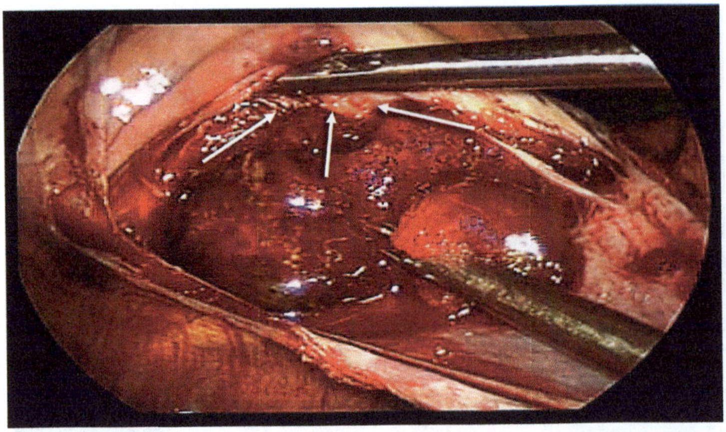

Fig. 7.25: The basic of the tumor has been identified. With the long knife and/or the scissors the tissue can be removed in toto from the atrial wall.

7.5.2 Practical performing

In cases with a small tumor it is normally simple to demonstrate the situation. The blade used for the atrial hook should be shorter than for mitral valve repair because of the fact that a large part of the septum has to be seen. After introducing the blade and lifting up the atrial septum the stem of the tumor has to be identified clearly. In an optimal situation the stem is fixed at first with the forceps and then, using a long knife or the curved scissors, the tumor is removed *in toto* with epicardial tissue (▶Fig. 7.25).

Especially in cases with the tumor stem at the atrial septum, a tissue defect results from cutting out. It appears to be an atrial septal defect and has to be closed accordingly. This means that for small defects a direct suture will be used and for a larger one the implantation of a pericardial patch may be necessary. It seems to be important for these cases that the optical system includes a 30° scope to have a clear view to the structures shown above.

Tumors localized in the left ventricle are sometimes difficult to identify. The main reason is the morphology of papillary muscles with gaps and spaces behind. Between the single parts of the muscles and the chords the tumors may be hidden and in some cases it takes time to find them. For a better overview and a more effective searching of tumors, the use of leaflet hooks may be helpful (for details see Section 3.2). In cases of intraventricular tumors the advantage of an operation technique based on an optical system is clearly shown.

Once the tumor is found, the same procedure as for the atrial tumor can be carried out. If there is a part of a papillary muscle included into the tumor tissue or the complete cutting out needs the cut of a chord, a repair of the affected leaflet part may be necessary. The described techniques for implantation of Neochords will be used (see Section 5.5).

Atrial or left ventricular tumors are normally rare. For an explantation of an atrial tumo,r the wall part with the basic of the tumor must be cut out. A possible defect may be closed directly or by implantation of a patch.

Index

Printed and bound by CPI Group (UK) Ltd, Croydon, CR0 4YY
13/09/2026
14960855-0002